International Agency For Research On Cancer

The International Agency for Research on Cancer (IARC) was established in 1965 by the World Health Assembly, as an independently financed organization within the framework of the World Health Organization. The headquarters of the Agency are in Lyon, France.

The Agency conducts a programme of research concentrating particularly on the epidemiology of cancer and the study of potential carcinogens in the human environment. Its field studies are supplemented by biological and chemical research carried out in the Agency's laboratories in Lyon and, through collaborative research agreements, in national research institutions in many countries. The Agency also conducts a programme for the education and training of personnel for cancer research.

The publications of the Agency contribute to the dissemination of authoritative information on different aspects of cancer research. A complete list is printed at the back of this book. Information about IARC publications, and how to order them, is also available via the Internet at: **http://www.iarc.fr/**

International Union Against Cancer

The International Union Against Cancer (UICC) is a non-governmental organization devoted exclusively to all aspects of the worldwide fight against cancer. Founded in 1933, it now has 254 member organizations in 84 countries, including cancer leagues and societies, cancer research and/or treatment centres and, in certain countries, ministries of health. It carries out a wide range of programmes in collaboration with hundreds of volunteer experts in various cancer-related fields. The UICC is non-profit-making, non-political, and non-sectarian; its headquarters are in Geneva, Switzerland.

'Europe Against Cancer' Programme Of The Commission Of The European Communities

The 'Europe Against Cancer' programme, which has been ongoing since 1986, is the response of the European Community to the fight against cancer. Initiatives have been taken, in collaboration with the various partners in the Member States, in cancer prevention, training of health personnel, information, health education and medical research.

Chemoprevention in Cancer Control

Edited by M. Hakama, V. Beral,
E. Buiatti, J. Faivre and D.M. Parkin

IARC Scientific Publications No. 136

International Agency for Research on Cancer,
Lyon, 1996

Published by the International Agency for Research on Cancer,
150 cours Albert Thomas, F-69372 Lyon cedex 08, France

Distributed by Oxford University Press, Walton Street, Oxford, UK OX2 6DP (Fax: +44 1865 267782) and in
the USA by Oxford University Press, 2001 Evans Road, Carey, NC 27513, USA (Fax: +1 919 677 1303).
All IARC publications can also be ordered directly from IARC*Press*
(Fax: +33 72 73 83 02; E-mail: press@iarc.fr).

IARC Library Cataloguing in Publication Data

Chemoprevention in cancer control/
       editors, M. Hakama ... [et al.]

       (IARC Scientific Publication; 136)
       1. Antineoplastic agents – therapeutic use
       2. Neoplasms – drug therapy
       3. Neoplasms – prevention and control
       I. Hakama, M. II. Series

ISBN 92 832 2136 2   (NLM Classification: QZ 200)
ISSN 0300–5085

Foreword

The genesis of this volume lay in the need perceived by the Europe Against Cancer Programme of the European Union to have a review of the current state of knowledge concerning cancer chemoprevention, in order to guide its recommendations concerning public policy, and the commissioning of research studies in Europe. The proposal to achieve this through a workshop and an associated publication was made by the UICC (through its Committee on Evaluation of Prevention Programmes) and the IARC, in 1993. The objective of the Workshop was to bring together leading experts to review the results of recent empirical studies on the effectiveness of chemopreventive agents on the reduction of cancer risk. The topics selected were intended to cover the main areas of research in this field over the last 5–10 years, as well as important issues concerning the design of research studies, cost-effectiveness of chemoprevention, and ethical concerns. The discussions of the presentations by the participants were brought together by the editorial group in a set of conclusions and recommendations, which we hope will meet the original objectives of providing a guide to formulating future public health policy and research strategy.

P. Kleihues
Director, IARC

S. Tominaga
Chairman, Epidemiology Prevention Programme UICC

R. Kroes
Member of the High-level Committee of Cancer Experts of the Europe Against Cancer Programme; Chairman, Sub-Committee on Prevention

List of participants

UICC, IARC and EU Workshop on Chemoprevention and Cancer
Lyon, 18–19 January 1995

V. Beral
The Radcliffe Infirmary
Gibson Building
Oxford OX2 6HE
United Kingdom

E. Buiatti
Epidemiology Unit
Registro Tumori Toscano
Via S. Salvi, 12
I-50135 Florence, Italy

A. Costa
European School of Oncology
Via Ripamonti 435
I-20141 Milan, Italy

X. Castellsagué
Servei D'Epidemiologia I
Registre del Càncer
Hospital Duran I Reynals
Autovia Castelldefels, km. 2.7
E-08907 L'Hospitalet del
Llobregat, Spain

J. Cuzick
Department of Mathematics
Imperial Cancer Research
Fund, P.O. Box No. 123
Lincoln's Inn Fields
London WC2A 3PX
United Kingdom

N.E. Day
MRC Biostatistics Unit
Institute of Public Health
University Forvie Site
Robinson Way
Cambridge CB2 2SR
United Kingdom

J. Estebaranz
DGV/F/1 Europe Against
Cancer Programme -
'Cancer' Sector
Bât. J. Monnet - JMO C3/60
Plateau du Kirchberg
L-2920 Luxemburg
Luxemburg

J. Faivre
Registre Bourguignon du
Cancer Digestif

Faculté de Médecine
7, Boulevard Jeanne-D'Arc
F-21033 Dijon,
France

J.M. Gaziano
Division of Preventive
Medicine, Brigham and
Women's Hospital
900 Commonwealth Ave. East
Boston, MA 02215, USA

A. Green
Queensland Institute of
Medical Research
The Bancroft Centre
P.O. Royal Brisbane Hospital
Brisbane, Queensland 4029
Australia

J.D.F. Habbema
Erasmus Universiteit
Rotterdam, Postbus 1738
NL-3000 DR Rotterdam
The Netherlands

M. Hakama
Department of Public Health
University of Tampere
Box 607, SF-33101 Tampere,
Finland

J.K. Huttunen
Kansanterveyslaitos
Mannerheimintie 166
SF-00300 Helsinki, Finland

R. Joseph
EPIDAURE, CRLC-Centre
Val d'Aurelle,
F-34094 Montpellier cedex 5
France

R. Kroes
Rijksinstituut voor
Volksgezondheid en
Millieuhygiene, Antonie van
Leeuwenhoeklaan 9
NL-3720 BA Bilthoven
The Netherlands

M. Lipkin
Memorial Sloan-Kettering

Cancer Center
1275 York Avenue
New York, NY 10021
USA

D. Malvy
Laboratoire de Santé
Publique, Faculté de
Médecine, B.P. 3223
F-37032 Tours cedex
France

F.L. Meyskens, Jr.
Clinical Cancer Center,
University of California,
Irvine Medical Center,
101 The City Drive, Rt. 81,
Bldg. 23, Orange,
CA 92668, USA

P.P. Nair
Human Nutrition Research
Centre Bldg. 308,
10300 Baltimore Ave,
Beltsville, MD 20705, USA

G.S. Omenn
School of Public Health and
Community Medicine
University of Washington
Seattle, WA 98195
USA

U. Pastorino
Royal Brompton Hospital,
Sydney Street
London SW3 6NP
United Kingdom

D. Patrick
Fred Hutchinson Cancer
Research Center
Division of Public Health
Sciences, 1730 Minor
Avenue MP-201, Seattle,
WA 98101, USA

R. Peto
University of Oxford
Clinical Trial Services Unit
Radcliffe Infirmary
Oxford OX2 6HE
United Kingdom

H. Sancho-Garnier
EPIDAURE, CRLC-Centre
Val d'Aurelle,
F-34094 Montpellier cedex 5,
France

B.W. Stewart
Children's Leukaemia &
Cancer Research Centre
The Prince of Wales
Children's Hospital,
Randwick Sydney, NSW
2031, Australia

S. Tominaga
Aichi Cancer Center
Research Institute
1-1 Kanokoden,
Chikusa-ku
Nagoya 464, Japan

A. Turnbull
UICC
3 rue du Conseil-Général
CH-1205 Genève
Switzerland

U. Veronesi
European School of
Oncology,
Via Ripamonti 435
I-20141 Milan 1, Italy

IARC Participants

J. Estève
R. Kaaks
P. Kleihues
C. Malaveille
D. McGregor
H. Møller
R. Montesano
N. Muñoz
H. Ohshima
M.D. Parkin
B. Pignatelli
P. Pisani
R. Sankaranarayanan
R. Saracci
A. Sasco
J. Wilbourn
C. Wild
H. Yamasaki

Contents

Why chemoprevention?

M. Hakama

The question posed in the title 'why chemoprevention?' can be approached from two points of view. One can present the scientific background for chemopreventive actions, or one can ask whether chemoprevention is an appropriate way to control cancer, whether it is acceptable. The first approach is a question of facts, the other is a question of values. This paper places emphasis on the first. However, the second is also important and should influence both research and the practice of cancer control.

The scientific background
Dietary studies

The major impetus for cancer control through chemopreventive actions stems from studies on diet and cancer. Epidemiological classification into ecological studies, case–control studies and cohort studies will be used in the following for reasons of reliability and because of differences in the effects estimated by these studies.

The earliest studies were ecological: they were based on populations as observational units. Migrant studies are a powerful tool with which to demonstrate the influence of the environment on the risk of cancer. In the early 1960s, Haenszel & Segi (1) showed that migrants from Japan to the United States had a trend in stomach cancer mortality from high-risk in Japan to low-risk in the United States. The reverse was true for colon cancer: the originally low-risk Japanese migrants reached the high rates common in the United States within two generations. Because Haenszel & Segi could identify the first (Issei) and second generation (Nisei) migrants, they were able to show that the transition was more rapid for colorectal cancer than for stomach cancer (Fig. 1). Later, Bjelke (2) confirmed the results on the basis of Norwegian immigrants to the United States. The changes were obviously due to environmental exposures, most probably dietary habits, which were grossly different in Japan, Europe and the United States.

The other group of ecological studies was based on geographical differences and the correlation of these differences with the consumption of food items such as meat, potatoes, flour, fat, fish and vegetables in different countries. Very high correlations were identified. In fact, the correlations between colon cancer and meat consumption, breast cancer and fat intake (3), and stomach cancer and consumption of cereals used as flour (4) were as high as the ecological correlations between lung cancer and smoking of cigarettes (5), one of the strongest dose–response relationships in cancer epidemiology.

Several dietary items correlate with cancer risk (6, 7). Fruits and vegetables show, quite consistently, a protective effect on cancer risk. In their review of case–control studies, Steinmetz & Potter (8) found that 87% of the studies on raw and fresh vegetables showed a protective effect, as did 61% of the studies on raw and fresh fruit (Table 1). Carrots were of special interest in many of the case–control studies, because of the high levels of β-carotene. In a review of 34 studies on the effect of carrots, Steinmetz & Potter reported that 27 of them showed a protective effect on cancer risk.

The large cohort studies in Japan (9), Norway (10) and the United States (8, 11) confirmed that the high and frequent consumption of fruits and vegetables was consistently correlated with a low risk of cancer (Table 2). However, the magnitude of the effect was twofold or less and it fell short of the relative risk of 10 between smoking and lung cancer. This was contrary to what one would have expected on the basis of ecological studies.

Studies on blood biochemistry and cancer

A greater amount of direct evidence on the specific causes of cancer can be obtained through the analysis of the levels of chemical substances in the body, particularly in the blood, than can be obtained on the basis of dietary data. Such research also provides an insight into the mechanisms by which the consumption of food may cause or protect against cancer. It has been suggested that biochemical substances, such as carotenoids, vitamins C and E, folic acid, selenium and other trace elements, can reduce the risk of cancer (6, 12).

High levels of blood carotenoid and retinol were relatively consistently associated in different studies with a low risk of cancer (13, 14, 15, 16). The prospective studies showed a stronger association between β-carotene and the risk of lung cancer, stomach cancer and cancers at several other anatomical sites than between blood retinol and these risks.

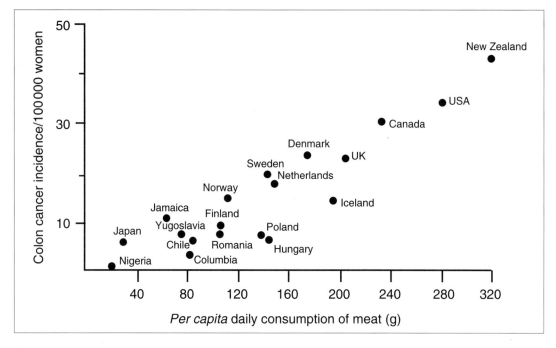

Fig. 1. Correlation between colon cancer incidence in various countries and meat consumption (redrawn from *3*). 'These striking age-standardized correlations do not necessarily suggest that either meat or some type of fat are major determinants of either colon or breast cancer, but they do suggest that manipulable determinants of these cancers do exist' (*3*).

A high intake of vitamin C was associated with a low risk of cancer. In a review, Block (*17*) found that 33 out of 46 studies showed a statistically significant inverse association. The effect was strongest for cancers in aerodigestive organs.

The trace elements have been the subject of less intensive epidemiological research. There is evidence that dietary selenium protects against cancer (*18*). In 10 out of 13 cohort studies based on serum sample banks, low levels of selenium were associated with a high risk of cancer (*19*).

Several biochemical substances were measured in the serum sample study on 60 000 people in Finland (*19*). The samples originated from the Social Insurance Insitution of Finland, which carried out a mobile clinic health survey during 1968–1972. The data were linked to the Finnish Cancer Registry. In the period between acquiring the sample and 1977, altogether 864 cases of cancer were diagnosed. A nested, 1:2 matched case–control study was carried out, and retinol, retinol-binding protein, β-carotene, α-tocopherol, selenium and ceruloplasmin were analysed. The relative risks by quintiles were, as a

rule, less than 2, and none of them was statistically significant for women (Tables 3 and 4).

In general, there seems to be an inverse relationship between the specificity of the hypothesis studied and the strength of the association. The ecological studies, whether based on a correlation between food consumption and cancer risk in different countries or on migrant studies, imply a very strong correlation. At an individual level, there is a relatively strong correlation between dietary items and cancer risk, but not as strong as was expected on the basis of ecological observations. If anything, the correlation is even less when the epidemiological studies on individuals are based on levels of biochemical substances in the body. In principle, one expects a reverse order in the strength of the association, because the hypotheses based on biochemistry are more specific than those based on the relatively broad dietary items, and more specific still than those based on the ecological observations of large populations.

The final proof of the causal effect is by means of randomized experiments. There are preventive

Table 1. Number of case–control studies on diet and cancer showing a protective effect of selected dietary items (8)

Dietary item	Number of studies	% Showing protective effect
Raw or fresh vegetables	15	87
Leafy green vegetables	43	74
Raw or fresh fruit	18	61
Carrots	34	79

Table 2. Relative risk of cancer among users of vegetables and fruits in selected cohort studies

Study	Site	Vegetables	Fruits
Norway (10)	Lung	0.5	0.7
Japan (9)	All	0.7	–
US (11)	Lung	0.8	0.6
US Iowa (8,12)	Lung	0.5	0.8

trials currently ongoing to evaluate the efficacy of chemoprevention. Because of the limitations of, and inconsistencies in, the epidemiological evidence so far, such trials are urgently needed.

Is chemoprevention the right approach to control?

Chemoprevention also has an ethical dimension. First, it seems that the scientific evidence on the effectiveness of chemoprevention may not be sufficient for large-scale programmes or for a general public health policy.

Even if such evidence was available, the problem of finding the means of prevention would remain. In principle, both regulative actions and health education of individuals are available methods. Fluoridation of the water supply is an example of regulation of the level of exposure that provoked discussion. In Finland, selenium was added to fertilizers, and in this way, low levels of selenium intake were increased to meet international standards. The protests in Finland were minimal, but some experts in other countries regarded the activity as ethically questionable.

Chemoprevention using pills and capsules could make up deficiencies in the diet. A basic question that follows from this is whether it is as acceptable to supplement diet using products of the pharmaceutical industry as it is to influence healthy eating habits in the society. First, the effect on health of supplementation with a single agent or various selected agents is not fully understood. Secondly, and more broadly, eating or dietary practices are also a mixture of sociocultural habits. They may change quite unintentionally in such a way that the final outcome of supplementation is not beneficial either to health or, more broadly, to the well-being of the individual from the psycho-social point of view.

An alternative to chemoprevention is modification of diet. Some individuals may be more interested in the culinary aspects of a food item than in its

Table 3. Smoking-adjusted relative risks of total cancer by quintiles of serum vitamin and selenium levels among men: The Cancer Registry follow-up of the Mobile Clinic Health Survey in Finland 1968–1977 (24)

Substance	Quintile (highest to lowest)					P-Value for trend
	1	2	3	4	5	
Retinol	1.0	1.0	1.1	1.2	1.4	0.02
Retinol-binding protein	1.0	1.3	1.3	1.2	1.7	0.06
β-Carotene	1.0	0.9	1.5	1.1	1.3	0.01
α-Tocopherol	1.0	1.0	1.5	1.6	1.3	0.03
Selenium	1.0	1.2	1.5	1.8	2.4	0.001

Table 4. Smoking-adjusted relative risks of total cancer by quintiles of serum vitamin and selenium levels among women: The Cancer Registry follow-up of the Mobile Clinic Health Survey in Finland 1968–1977 (24)

| Substance | Quintile (highest to lowest) | | | | | P-Value for trend |
	1	2	3	4	5	
Retinol	1.0	1.2	1.2	1.5	1.5	0.08
Retinol-binding protein	1.0	1.0	0.9	1.2	1.2	0.21
β-Carotene	1.0	0.9	1.1	1.3	1.0	0.26
α-Tocopherol	1.0	0.9	1.1	1.1	1.7	0.08
Selenium	1.0	1.1	1.3	1.0	1.2	0.60

carcinogeneity. The replacement of dietary items with pharmacological products removes the social or culinary dimension of a meal.

As is often the case in medicine, improvement in the quality of life and an increase in the length of life may be the competing outcomes of alternative interventions. Balancing the effects on different dimensions of life involves value judgements. Therefore, chemoprevention is not only a question of facts but also one of values. The workshop and this monograph focus on the facts, but at the same time the question of values is also considered.

Purpose of this monograph

Diet and nutrition are important causes of cancer. The classical estimate is that one-third of cancers are caused by diet. Doll & Peto (3) emphasized 15 years ago that this estimate is subject to substantial uncertainty and that the dietary habits and substances that cause cancer are largely unknown.

Since that time, methods have improved and knowledge has increased. Specifically, the large cohort studies based on serum sample banks have investigated the causative effects of relatively specific

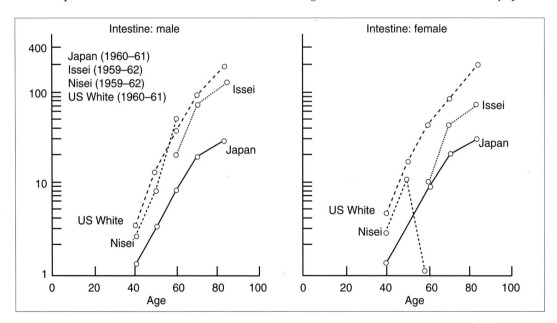

Fig. 2. Age-specific death rates from cancer of the large intestine among Japanese, Japanese migrants in the US, and the US white population (1).

substances. On the basis of epidemiological results and other evidence, several preventive trials on chemopreventive agents have been started. The purpose of the background workshop and this monograph is to give a state-of-the-art overview on the experimental evidence, based on preventive randomized trials on humans, concerning the effectiveness of chemoprevention in reducing the risk of cancer.

The UICC has been active in evaluating interventions, both screening and primary prevention programmes (20, 21). One of the activities that has been given priority by IARC is chemoprevention (22). The EU programme 'Europe Against Cancer' has shown an interest in chemoprevention (23). This monograph is the result of these different efforts and interests. The aim of the monograph is to collate information concerning the preventive trials of the effectiveness of chemoprevention in reducing the risk of cancer, and to discuss the merits and deficiencies of such studies.

References

1 Haenszel W, Segi M. Stomach cancer among the Japanese. In: Harris RJC, ed. *Proceedings of the 9th International Cancer Congress, Panels*. Heidelberg, Springer-Verlag, 1967:55–63 (UICC Monograph Series, Vol. 10).

2 Bjelke E. Epidemiologic studies of cancer of the stomach, colon, and rectum, with special emphasis on the role of diet. Abstracts and Literature Review. *Scand J Gastroenterol*, 1974, 9:1–235.

3 Doll R, Peto R. *The causes of cancer*. Oxford, Oxford University Press, 1981.

4 Hakama M, Saxen EA. Cereal consumption and gastric cancer. *Int J Cancer*, 1967, 2:265–268.

5 Peto R, Lopez A, Boreham J, Thun M, Heath C, *Mortality from smoking in developed countries 1950–2000*. Oxford University Press, 1994.

6 Mettlin CJ, Aoki K, eds. *Recent progress in research on nutrition and cancer*. New York, Wiley-Liss, 1990 (Progress in Clinical and Biological Research, Vol. 346).

7 Greenwald P, Clifford C. Dietary prevention. In: Greenwald P, Kramer BS, Weed DL, eds. *Cancer prevention and control*. New York, Marcel Dekker, Inc., 1995:302–327.

8 Steinmetz KA, Potter JD. Vegetables, fruit, and cancer. I. Epidemiology. *Cancer Causes and Control*, 1991, 2:325–357.

9 Hirayama T. *Life-style and mortality. A large-scale census-based cohort study in Japan*. Basel, Karger, 1990 (Contributions to Epidemiology and Biostatistics, Vol. 6).

10 Kvåle G, Bjelke E, Gart JJ. Dietary habits and lung cancer risk. *Int J Cancer*, 1983, 31:397–405.

11 de Long W, Hammond EC. Lung cancer, fruit, green salad and vitamin pills. *Chin Med J*, 1985, 98:206–210.

12 Steinmetz KA, Potter JD. Vegetables, fruit, and cancer. II. Mechanisms. *Cancer Causes and Control*, 1991, 2:427–442.

13 Fontham ETH. Protective dietary factors and lung cancer. *Int J Epidemiol*, 1990, 19:S32–S42.

14 Hennekens CH, Mayrent SL, Willet W. Vitamin A, carotenoids, and retinoids. *Cancer*, 1986, 58:1837–1841.

15 Willett WC. Vitamin A and lung cancer. *Nutr Rev*, 1990, 48:201–211.

16 Ziegler RG. A review of epidemiologic evidence that carotenoids reduce the risk of cancer. *J Nutr*, 1989, 119:116–122.

17 Block G. Vitamin C and cancer prevention: the epidemiologic evidence. *Am J Clin Nutr*, 1991, 53:270S–282S.

18 Willett WC. Selenium, vitamin E, fiber, and the incidence of human cancer: an epidemiologic perspective. *Adv Exp Med Biol*, 1986, 206:27–34.

19 Knekt P et al. Vitamin E and cancer prevention. *Am J Clin Nutr*, 1991, 53:283S–286S.

20 Miller AB et al., eds. *Cancer Screening*. Cambridge, Cambridge University Press, 1991.

21 Hakama M et al., eds. *Evaluating effectiveness of primary prevention of cancer*. Lyon, International Agency for Research on Cancer, 1990 (IARC Sci. Publ. No. 103).

22 Stewart BW. *An evaluation programme for cancer preventive agents*. Lyon, International Agency for Research on Cancer, 1995 (IARC Technical Report No. 23).

23 Buiatti E, Balzi D, Barchielli A. *Intervention trials of cancer prevention: Results and new research programmes*. Lyon, International Agency for Research on Cancer, 1994 (IARC Technical Report No. 18).

24 Hakama M et al. Linkage of serum sample bank and cancer registry in epidemiological studies. In: Mettlin CJ, Aoki K, eds. *Recent Progress in Research on Nutrition and Cancer*. New York, Wiley-Liss, 1990: 169–178.

M. Hakama
Tampere School of Public Health, University of Tampere, Box 607, FIN-33101 Tampere, Finland

Methodological issues in the design of primary prevention trials

J.M. Gaziano*, C.H. Hennekens and J.E. Buring

Careful consideration of the issues involved in the design and conduct of clinical trials is essential for valid results to be achieved. Specifically, if the trial is well designed with respect to timing, choice of study design and population, completeness of follow-up and compliance, size and duration, it can offer reliable evidence about the positive, negative or null effect of an intervention. With these considerations in mind, the Women's Health Study is being conducted among nearly 40 000 United States female health professionals over the age of 45 years, using a factorial design to test the roles of vitamin E, β-carotene and aspirin in the primary prevention of cancer and cardiovascular disease. This trial is a companion study to the Physicians' Health Study, a primary prevention trial testing the role of β-carotene in the primary prevention of cancer and cardiovascular disease. The ultimate goal of these methodological considerations is to design studies that can clearly prove or refute the hypotheses being tested.

Introduction

Advances in the diagnosis and treatment of cancer, as well as an increased understanding of the mechanisms of the disease, have provided, and will certainly continue to provide, enormous benefit to individuals affected. At the same time, interventions that may prevent common cancers from developing in healthy people could, at least in theory, afford even greater benefits to society as a whole. For example, a complete cure for leukaemia, which accounts for 18 000 of the approximately 540 000 total cancer deaths in the United States each year, would be a remarkable breakthrough in medical research. In terms of public health impact, however, the identification of a micronutrient supplement with the ability to reduce by even 15% the development of epithelial cell cancers, which account for 90% of cancer deaths in the United States, could conceivably prevent 73 000 cancer deaths annually.

*Correspondence: J.M. Gaziano, Division of Preventive Medicine, Brigham and Women's Hospital, 900 Commonwealth Avenue East, Boston, MA 02215-1204, USA.

In considering the design of any clinical trial, there are a number of major issues that must be addressed. These include the timing, the choice of the most efficient study design, completeness of follow-up, level of compliance, size of the likely risk reduction, and the availability of sufficient numbers of end-points. In this report, each of these will be discussed in the context of the United States Women's Health Study (WHS), a randomized, double-blind, placebo-controlled trial of vitamin E, β-carotene and aspirin in the primary prevention of cancer and cardiovascular disease among approximately 40 000 female health professionals in the United States (1, 2), which is in many ways based on our experience in the Physicians' Health Study (PHS), a randomized, placebo-controlled, double-blind primary prevention trial that was designed to test the risks and benefits of aspirin and β-carotene in the prevention of cancer and cardiovascular disease (3).

Timing of randomized trials

Perhaps the first issue that must be addressed by investigators planning a trial is when to undertake it. Although for any epidemiological study there must be a balance between evidence supporting the hypothesis being tested and the gap in knowledge or accepted practices, which may be filled by the results, achieving this balance is a particularly delicate matter for randomized clinical trials. For both ethical and practical reasons, there must be sufficient doubt about the agent or agents to be tested for treatment to be withheld from half the subjects, and at the same time there must be sufficient belief in the agent's potential to justify exposing the other half of the willing and eligible participants.

When work first began on the WHS, the hypothesis that aspirin prevents recurrence of myocardial infarction (MI) had been tested in numerous randomized secondary prevention studies among both men and women, but it had only been tested in a randomized primary prevention trial among men. The PHS had shown a significant 44% reduction in fatal and non-fatal MI among those given 325 mg of aspirin on alternate days, as compared with those on placebo (4, 5). The need to assess the risk and benefits of aspirin among women, who are at lower risk of cardiovascular disease, was clear.

The hypothesis that antioxidant vitamins might reduce cancer risk was perhaps the most promising of the hypotheses concerning inhibition of carcinogenesis by micronutrients. Many case–control and cohort studies provide remarkably consistent data suggesting that consumption of foods rich in these antioxidant vitamins reduces the risks of developing epithelial cancers originating in epithelial cells. These data raise the question of a possible role of antioxidants in primary prevention of cancer and cardiovascular disease. Unfortunately, no matter how consistent the observational data are, and no matter how much more data become available, they will never be able to provide a definitive answer to the question of the possible role of β-carotene or α-tocopherol in reducing cancer risks.

It seemed timely to conduct a randomized trial of β-carotene and vitamin E because of the rapid increase in supplementation with these micronutrients despite the lack of clear benefit. Even after adjustments for inflation, there has been a several-fold increase in sales of vitamin pills in the United States. A recent survey indicated that 64% of United States adults report regular multivitamin use, and 43% and 34% regularly take vitamins C and E, respectively. Thus the use of nutritional supplements was already widespread and seemed likely to continue to increase, even in the absence of reliable evidence concerning possible health benefits. It therefore seemed important to begin a trial of β-carotene and vitamin E among women as soon as possible, since a failure to do so might have made such a study unfeasible in the future.

The effects of micronutrients on the chemoprevention of cancer are extremely difficult to evaluate because they are likely to be small to moderate in size, of the order of a 10–30% reduction in risk. In observational epidemiological studies, effects of this magnitude may be similar in size to the effects of confounding. In such circumstances, randomized trials can yield the only direct evidence on which to base a judgement on the ability of a micronutrient to reduce cancer incidence. However, because of the logistic complexity and relatively high costs of randomized trials, it is essential that they are well designed, carefully conducted, and properly analysed.

Design efficiency

With respect to the choice of the best and most efficient study design, one approach that is gaining in popularity is the use of a factorial design, a technique which improves efficiency by testing two or more hypotheses simultaneously (6). In the WHS, a 2 × 2 × 2 factorial design is being employed. The 40 000 participants are being randomly assigned to two groups, one taking aspirin and the other taking an aspirin placebo. Each of these groups is further divided into two subgroups, taking either β-carotene or a β-carotene placebo. Each of these groups is then further subdivided into two, one taking vitamin E the other placebo. There will therefore be eight treatment arms. A participant could thus be taking aspirin only, carotene only, vitamin E only, any combination of the three agents, or all placebos. The principal advantage of this type of design is its ability to answer two or more questions in a single trial for only a marginal increase in cost. Moreover, the use of a factorial design can permit the testing of a less mature hypothesis, such as the role of antioxidants in cancer chemoprevention, together with a more mature hypothesis, such as the role of aspirin in cardiovascular disease, for which there is sufficient evidence available to justify mounting a large-scale investigation.

With respect to the study agents, antioxidants represent an attractive option for cancer chemoprevention. First, they provide the ability to study a single dietary component in isolation. Second, antioxidant vitamins are available in pill form. This allows for easy delivery of the study intervention. In addition, a placebo can be manufactured easily, aiding in the blinding of the study. These micronutrients also have a favourable side-effect profile which enhances compliance. Finally, if antioxidant vitamins prove to be effective, their use would not be restricted to high-risk individuals, because of the low side-effects, and they could be safely recommended to the entire population. β-carotene and vitamin E are two abundant and widely available dietary antioxidants and considerable observational data suggest that these dietary components may reduce the risks of cardiovascular disease and cancer.

We have chosen the natural form of α-tocopherol. The synthetic preparation is composed of eight stereoisomers, only one of which (RRR) is available in nature. Recent data suggest that the natural form is preferentially incorporated into circulating lipoproteins and body tissues. There is a clear discrimination between the naturally occurring RRR stereoisomer of α-tocopherol and the synthetic SRR stereoisomer (7). Both isomers appear to be absorbed via the gut and secreted into chylomicrons, however the RRR form is preferentially incorporated into circulating LDL for delivery to the peripheral tissues at a ratio of the natural RRR isomer to the synthetic SRR isomer of 2:1. Accumulation in various tissue revealed a ratio of RRR to SRR as high as 5:1 (7, 8). Tissue levels appear to be critical for disease prevention in certain animal models (9). One site of discrimination appears to be a specific hepatic protein which is responsible for the incorporation of α-tocopherol into lipoprotein particles, and cytosolic transport proteins have been identified in other tissues.

β-carotene, the most common dietary carotenoid, is found in high concentrations in many fresh fruits and vegetables such as carrots, squash, melons, spinach and broccoli. β-carotene has the ability to quench singlet oxygen and is a chain-breaking antioxidant. It exists as several different isomers in nature, including all-*trans*, 9-*cis*, 13-*cis* and 15-*cis* isomers. Bioavailability studies suggest that the all-*trans* isomer of β-carotene is preferentially incorporated into circulating lipids for delivery to peripheral tissues after chronic supplementation (10). We are using the synthetic preparation of β-carotene due to its predominant all-*trans* content.

Completeness of follow-up

The third point to keep in mind when designing a trial is the need to obtain complete follow-up on all participants. This is one of the major issues involved in ensuring that the results of a study will be valid, and is accepted as such throughout the scientific community. A trial that enrolled 30 000 people initially but collected follow-up data from only 20 000 people 5 years later may not produce an interpretable result. Thus, it is essential to choose a study population consisting of people from whom complete information can be obtained over an extended period of time. In this regard, it is important to keep in mind that if complete follow-up data on all randomized patients are not possible, any follow-up data – at the very least, vital status – is better than none.

Careful selection of the population for a trial can be a great asset in achieving high levels of both compliance and follow-up. The choice of health

professionals for the WHS study population was made for a number of ethical, scientific and logistic reasons. From a practical point of view, our previous studies showed that the collaboration of health professionals would result in excellent compliance with their assigned regimens as well as the receipt of completed questionnaires. This allowed the trial to be conducted entirely by mail at a small fraction of the usual cost for intervention studies. Specifically, previous trials of primary prevention in the United States have generally been conducted in hospitals, clinics or laboratories, and the participants seen periodically by physicians or other health professionals. In such studies, costs have ranged from $3000 to over $15 000 per randomized subject. In contrast, total costs in the WHS are approximately $100 per year of follow-up. Finally, health professionals are easier to follow than members of the general population, thus increasing the likelihood that complete morbidity and mortality data would be collected on all participants for the duration of the trial.

While limiting participation to a special group, such as health professionals, has the above-described advantages, one major disadvantage is worth mentioning. It may not be possible to generalize the result to a broader population who may be less healthy or less compliant with the intervention. Despite this concern over the ability to extrapolate the result, the selection of this special population provided an enhanced opportunity to establish a causal relation, if one exits, at a very low cost.

Level of compliance

An issue closely related to follow-up is the need to maintain high compliance with the study regimens. The reason for the very strong emphasis on maintaining high compliance and follow-up in a trial relates to the fact that the inclusion in the analyses of data on all participants, regardless of compliance or drop-out status, is essential, since the only truly randomized comparison in a trial is between the total treatment group and the total placebo group. Such a comparison is the most valid, because of the unique properties of randomization. First, in a large sample, the random allocation of treatments will virtually ensure an equal distribution of all known confounders. While it is possible to achieve control of known confounders in observational studies, only randomized trials have the ability to control confounders that are present but cannot be easily measured or have not yet been identified. This degree of control of both known and unknown confounding provides a level of assurance about the validity of the data from a randomized trial that is simply not possible with other study designs.

The danger of restricting the analysis only to those who are compliant with the study regimen relates to the fact that those who are willing and able to comply fully with any given treatment regimen are only a selected subgroup of the total study population. It is likely that such subjects differ from the other participants in ways that might affect their ultimate response to the treatment. This can best be illustrated by the experience of the Coronary Drug Project in their trial of clofibrate in the prevention of mortality after myocardial infarction. In this randomized, double-blind, placebo-controlled trial, 1103 patients were given clofibrate while 2789 were given placebo. When all randomized subjects were included in the main analysis of the trial, the 5-year total mortality rates in the two groups were 20% and 20.9% (11). To explore the effect of compliance on this outcome, the investigators then analysed the mortality experience within the clofibrate group and found that those whose compliance was at least 80% had a mortality rate of 15%, compared with 24.6% among those who were poor compliers. While such a finding might seem to suggest that clofibrate itself actually does reduce mortality, a similar analysis within the placebo group found a comparable disparity in mortality between compliers and non-compliers, with rates of 15.1% and 28.2%, respectively. These differences between compliers and non-compliers were unchanged after the control of 40 known possible confounders through multiple logistic regression analysis. These data show very clearly that compliers are different from non-compliers in ways that affect their prognosis. If it seems useful or interesting to assess differences in outcomes among compliers only, an additional analysis can be performed, as was done in the Coronary Drug Project. However, a restricted analysis should not substitute for a full analysis of all randomized patients.

A strategy we use to enhance compliance is a run-in period for all subjects prior to actual randomization. We have enrolled over 66 000 initially willing and eligible female health professionals in the run-in phase. Participants take their daily pills from calendar packs containing aspirin placebo, β-carotene placebo and vitamin E placebo. We chose to use placebos in the run-in for two main reasons. First, we anticipated low side-effects from all the agents. A run-in is sometimes employed to eliminate those who cannot comply with an intervention due to side-effects, but since there are few side-effects for the study agents, this would not result in substantial non-compliance once subjects were given active agents. Second, we wanted to test for side-effects of each agent in the trial, something that we would not have had the opportunity to do if we had eliminated those with side-effects to either of the active agents during the run-in. In addition, the possible beneficial effects from β-carotene and vitamin E are cumulative and the side-effects are minimal, so that it was optimal not to expose the entire cohort to an active drug before randomization. After approximately 3 months, we sent the participants questionnaires, and individuals who reported side-effects, the development of an exclusion criterion or a desire to discontinue participation, and even those who wished to continue but whose compliance we deemed inadequate, were excluded from the trial before randomization.

The use of a run-in period allowed for the implementation of an additional strategy to enhance the sensitivity of the trial: the collection of pre-randomization blood specimens from participating health professionals. Analyses of blood specimens for baseline levels of carotenoids and tocopherols may permit the identification of particular subgroups of participants, if any, that stand to benefit most from dietary supplementation with β-carotene. Specifically, a trial among 40 000 health professionals would easily demonstrate a 30% reduction in total epithelial cancer incidence related to β-carotene or vitamin E, if such an effect exists, but would not have sufficient power to detect a significant difference between treatment groups if the overall effect were only 10%. It is possible, however, that a small but important 10% overall reduction in cancer incidence could result from a much larger effect confined exclusively to that subgroup of women who had low carotene or retinol levels at entry. This important public health finding could easily be detected, given the ability to stratify participants by baseline levels of these parameters, and future public health intervention could be aimed at that particular subgroup.

Previous studies indicated that, on the whole, health professionals were willing and able to provide processed specimens, and in fact viewed the request as enhancing the scientific quality of the WHS. In the PHS, as a result of these efforts, blood samples were received from 14 916 randomized physicians. Blood sample collection rates are comparable in the WHS.

Size of risk reduction

The fourth question that needs to be considered in designing a prevention trial is how to obtain a large enough reduction in risk to be able to detect it accurately and reliably. This consideration is of particular relevance to cancer trials, where long latency periods may delay the emergence of a protective effect for several years. Thus, to detect a large enough relative risk estimate with adequate power, it is imperative to plan a sufficient duration of treatment and follow-up.

Sufficient end-points

Finally, we have to consider how to accumulate a sufficient number of events that are considered as end-points to test the hypothesis adequately. In designing trials, investigators often focus efforts on increasing the size of the study population. However, the effective sample size of a trial is proportional not to the number of individuals enrolled, but rather to the number of events they experience that are classified as end-points. An adequate number of events is necessary but not sufficient to test a chemopreventive hypothesis adequately. The end-points must occur sufficiently long after the initiation of the intervention. For example, it would be far preferable to follow a cohort of 20 000 individuals for 15 years than to follow one of 150 000 participants for 2 years, even if similar numbers of end-points accrued in both cohorts.

The length of the planned follow-up period of a trial should always take into account the possibility that the actual rate of accrual of end-points may be less than projected, since whose who enrol in trials seem to have lower mortality than those who are eligible but who do not enrol, regardless of the hypotheses being tested and even regardless of treatment assignment. In the PHS, for example, the number of cardiovascular deaths experienced by the randomized participants was considerably less than is expected among a general population of white males of the same age distribution in the United States. Further, there may be secular changes in mortality, such as occurred in the Multiple Risk Factor Intervention Trial (MRFIT; 12), where the entire United States population experienced a 3% per annum decline in cardiovascular mortality during the 1970s (13). Thus, lower than expected event rates are not uncommon in clinical trials and can produce a null result that is uninformative. However, since end-points accumulate exponentially rather than arithmetically as the population ages, simply extending the duration of the study can achieve statistical significance of an effect.

In addition to making the follow-up period long enough, a second strategy to accumulate sufficient end-points is to select a high-risk population. In the case of chronic diseases, an important criterion for this choice is age. Since end-points accumulate exponentially with increasing age, the effect of this factor on the number of end-points can be dramatic. For example, in a study of cancer, a population of 10 000 men aged 40–55 years would contribute only a fraction of the deaths which would accumulate among a similar group of men aged 65 or older. On the other hand, the size of the relative risk for a given exposure may decrease at older ages. Clearly, in selecting the optimum study population and sample size for any given trial, scientific considerations must be balanced with issues of feasibility and costs.

Conclusions

The effectiveness of all these strategies can be illustrated by looking at the compliance and follow-up rates among those randomized in the PHS (1, 2). After an average of 11.7 years of follow-up, 81% of randomized subjects were still taking β-carotene or its placebo. The validity of these self-reported compliance figures has been supported by analyses of blood samples for blood levels of β-carotene obtained from a sample of participants. With respect to obtaining complete follow-up information from all participants, after 11.7 years of follow-up, morbidity follow-up is 99% complete and mortality follow-up is 100% complete. Thus, to date, not a single participant has been lost to follow-up. Both these compliance and follow-up results are exceptionally high, reflecting very gratifying levels of cooperation among the participating physicians. Preliminary data suggest that compliance and follow-up rates will be comparable in the WHS.

In conclusion, the ultimate goal of all the methodological choices mentioned is to allow a trial clearly to refute or to prove the hypotheses that are being tested. Large-scale randomized trials, such as the PHS and WHS, that can be conducted at a low cost per participant are necessary to advance knowledge concerning possible cancer chemoprevention agents in the general population. However, only those with adequate methodological rigour should be carried out. Each trial must be designed and conducted in such a way that it can obtain either a definitive positive or negative result on which public policy can be based, or a null result that is truly informative, which will then safely permit the rechannelling of already limited resources to other areas of research.

References

1 Buring JE, Hennekens CH. The Women's Health Study: Summary of the study design. *J Myocard Ischemia*, 1992, 4:27–29.

2 Buring JE, Hennekens CH. The Women's Health Study: Rationale and background. *J Myocard Ischemia*, 1992, 4:30–40.

3 Hennekens CH, Eberlein KA, for the Physicians' Health Study Research Group. A Randomized Trial of Aspirin and Beta-Carotene among U.S. Physicians. *Prev Med*, 1985, 14:165–168.

4 Steering Committee of the Physicians' Health Study. Preliminary Report: Findings from the aspirin component of the ongoing Physicians' Health Study. *N Engl J Med*, 1988, 318:262–264.

5 Steering Committee of the Physicians' Health Study. Final report on the aspirin component of the ongoing Physicians' Health Study. *N Engl J Med*, 1989, 321:129–135.

6 Stampfer MJ et al. The 2 × 2 factorial design: Its application to a randomized trial of aspirin and beta-carotene in U.S. physicians. *Stat Med*, 1985, 4:111–116.

7 Ingold KU et al. Biokinetics of and Discrimination Between Dietary RRR- and SRR- α-Tocopherols in the Male Rat. *Lipids*, 1987, 22:163–172.

8 Traber MG et al. RRR- and SRR-α-tocopherols are secreted without discrimination in human chylomicrons, but RRR α-tocopherol is preferentially secreted in very low density lipoproteins. *J Lipid Research*, 1990, 31:679–685

9 Keaney JF et al. Dietary antioxidants preserve endothelium-dependent vessel relaxation in rabbits. *Proc Natl Acad Sci*, 1993, 90:11 880–11 884.

10 Gaziano JM et al. Discrimination in absorption of beta carotene isomers following oral supplementation with either all-trans or 9-cis beta carotene. *Am J Clin Nutr*, 1995, 61:1218–1252.

11 Coronary Drug Project Research Group. Clofibrate and niacin in coronary heart disease. *J Am Med Assoc*, 1975, 231:360–381.

12 Multiple Risk Factor Intervention Trial Research Group (1982). Risk factor changes and morbidity results). *JAMA*, 248:1465–1477.

13 Havlik RJ, Feinleib M, eds. *Proceedings of the Conference on the Decline in Coronary Heart Disease Mortality*. US, DHEW, NIH Publication No. 79-1610. 1979.

J.M. Gaziano, C.H. Hennekens and J.E. Buring
Division of Preventive Medicine, Department of Medicine, Brigham and Women's Hospital and Harvard Medical School, Boston, MA, USA

J.E. Buring
Department of Ambulatory Care and Prevention, Harvard Medical School, Boston, MA, USA

J.M. Gaziano
Department of Medicine, Veteran's Affairs Medical Center, Brockton/West Roxbury, MA, USA; and Cardiovascular Division, Department of Medicine, Brigham and Women's Hospital and Harvard Medical School, Boston, MA, USA

C.H. Hennekens
Department of Ambulatory Care and Prevention, Harvard Medical School, Boston, MA, USA; and Department of Epidemiology, Harvard School of Public Health, Boston, MA, USA

Chemoprevention of cancers of the oral cavity and the head and neck

R. Sankaranarayanan*, B. Mathew, P.P. Nair, T. Somanathan, C. Varghese, R. Jyothirmayi and M. Krishnan Nair

Head and neck cancer, particularly oral cancer, provides an ideal model to investigate chemoprevention as a cancer control methodology. Head and neck carcinogenesis evolves as a multistep process characterized by field cancerization, as evidenced by molecular, histological and clinical findings, for example accumulation of genetic damage (e.g. p53 mutations, micronuclei), pathological changes such as hyperplasia/metaplasia/dysplasia in exposed epithelium, precancerous lesions such as leukoplakia, and a high frequency of second primaries in treated head and neck cancer patients. Natural analogues of vitamin A, such as retinyl palmitate, and synthetic analogues, such as isotretinoin, fenretinide and etretinate, have been more widely investigated for their potential to modulate the above changes/events than have other agents such as β-carotene and vitamin E. A variety of end-points, such as leukoplakia, loco-regional recurrence and second primary cancers, and intermediate end-points, such as micronuclei, have been used in these studies. Leukoplakia has been shown to regress with the use of retinoids, β-carotene and vitamin E; however, the lesions briskly recur once supplementation is stopped. Retinoids have been shown to prevent second primaries in treated head and neck cancer patients, although they were not found to be effective in preventing loco-regional recurrences of head and neck cancer. Synthetic retinoids were associated with significant toxicity, especially mucocutaneous reactions. Large studies are now ongoing to address whether long-term chemoprevention with retinoids, β-carotene and N-acetylcysteine reduces the incidence of second primary tumours in treated head and neck cancer patients. No intermediate end-point has so far been validated as a surrogate for cancer incidence. Nevertheless, they are useful in screening for chemopreventive agents and in monitoring compliance. In summary, retinoids seem to be significantly active in reversing oral leukoplakia.

*Correspondence: R. Sankaranarayanan
Unit of Descriptive Epidemiology, International Agency for Research on Cancer, 150 cours Albert Thomas, 69372 Lyon cedex 08, France

Long-term studies are required to address whether prolonged administration of retinoids would result in the reduction of head and neck cancer incidence and mortality rates in high-risk populations. Meanwhile, investigations should continue in order to identify and evaluate other effective and less toxic chemopreventive agents for head and neck cancer. Any attempt at chemoprevention of head and neck cancer should be undertaken within experimental settings only.

Introduction

Chemoprevention is currently being investigated as one of the methods of preventing head and neck epithelial cancers. Similarities in the aetiology, pathogenesis, natural history and anatomical relationships of head and neck cancer sites such as the oral cavity (ICD 140–145), oropharynx (ICD 146), hypopharynx (ICD 148–149) and larynx (ICD 161) have often led these diverse sites to be considered as a single group when discussing the preventive and therapeutic approaches to be used in their control.

Head and neck cancers are common in regions of the world where the smoking and chewing of tobacco and alcohol consumption are predominant habits among the population. These cancers accounted for an estimated 554 000 incident cases and 335 000 deaths in 1985 (1, 2). High incidence rates have been observed in south Asia (India, Pakistan, Bangladesh), the Pacific islands, Puerto Rico and certain regions of France and South America. The trends in the incidence and mortality suggest different patterns in different regions. For instance, in countries like India and Pakistan, a decline in chewing-related head and neck cancers, such as oral cancers and gingiva, and an increase in smoking-related cancers have been reported (3, 4). In Western countries, an increase in the incidence of and mortality from cancers of most head and neck subsites, particularly tongue and mouth cancers, has been observed in recent years (5).

Although primary prevention by tobacco control and moderation in alcohol should be the most successful strategy for the control of head and neck cancer, the evaluation of complementary approaches such as chemoprevention is important as a means of achieving and accelerating the pace of head and neck cancer control. Observations from animal studies and epidemiological investigations provide the biological basis of chemoprevention. Retinoids, carotenoids and vitamin E have blocked the progression of chemically induced oral carcinogenesis in animal studies and have resulted in the regression of hamster buccal pouch cancers (6, 7). Epidemiological studies have established the protective role of diets that are rich in fruits and vegetables in head and neck carcinogenesis, and the reduced risk of head and neck cancer associated with a high intake of vitamin A, vitamin E and carotenoids (8, 9, 10, 11, 12, 13, 14).

Head and neck cancer as an ideal model for chemoprevention

Head and neck carcinogenesis, particularly oral cancer, provides an ideal model to evaluate chemoprevention strategies. Head and neck cancers are an outcome of a multistep carcinogenic process that is conceptually divided into three phases: initiation, promotion and progression. Initiation involves an irreversible damage to DNA by carcinogens and, when this involves genes regulating cell growth and differentiation (e.g. tumour suppressor genes, proto-oncogenes), it may lead to the development of cancer. Promotion is the process by which the initiated cell is converted into a pre-neoplastic or cancerous cell. It is associated with the activation of proto-oncogenes and the inactivation of suppressor genes, leading to defects in differentiation, growth control and resistance to host immune response.

The various phases of carcinogenesis were highlighted by molecular, cytological, pathological and clinical studies of normal and premalignant/malignant tissues from high-risk subjects and head and neck cancer patients. The precancerous lesions, such as leukoplakia, submucous fibrosis, metaplasia and dysplasia, represent the promotion phase, and the *in situ* and invasive cancers represent the progression phase.

The clinical manifestations of head and neck carcinogenesis support the field cancerization concept, which assumes that the whole upper aerodigestive epithelial tract is prone to the carcinogenic process as a result of repeated exposure to carcinogens, and could undergo malignant transformation at various times (15). This is clearly demonstrated by the high frequency of second primary cancers in subjects with head and neck cancers (16, 17, 18, 19). According to the field cancerization theory, primary tumours and second primaries result from the progression of commonly initiated premalignant lesions.

The head and neck sites, in particular the oral cavity, are easily visible and accessible without the help of sophisticated equipment, and thus they have an advantage over other internal sites in that investigations and assessment of responses to chemoprevention are made easier.

Agents currently used in head and neck cancer chemoprevention and their mechanisms of action

Natural and synthetic analogues of vitamin A (retinoids), β-carotene, vitamin E , N-acetyl-l-cysteine (NAC) and selenium, and a naturally occurring blue-green alga, *Spirulina fusiformis*, feature among the reported studies of head and neck cancer chemoprevention. Retinoids are the most widely studied of all compounds; natural analogues such as retinyl palmitate/acetate and synthetic analogues such as 13-cis retinoic acid (13-cRA or isotretinoin), N-(4-hydroxyphenyl)-retinamide (4-HPR or fenretinide) and etretinate have been investigated. The mode of action of many chemopreventive agents is, for the most part, unclear. However, studies have identified certain properties which are relevant to chemoprevention. These are briefly discussed below.

Retinoids appear to exert their anticancer activity by their effect on cell differentiation, by stimulating immune cells that are depressed during carcinogenesis, and by inducing apoptosis, a programmed cell death (20, 21, 22, 23). Retinoids modulate the expression of a variety of genes involved in growth and differentiation, including genes encoding growth factors (e.g. PDGF, EGF, TGF-B), growth factor receptors (e.g. EGF-R, NGF-R), components of signal transduction (e.g. protein kinase C), proto-oncogenes (e.g. *myc*, *fos*), transcription factors and complementary cell surface and extracellular matrix adhesion molecules. It is likely that many retinol effects are mediated by its metabolic conversion to all transretinoic acid (RA). It is thought that nuclear retinoic acid receptors, which regulate gene expression, cell differentiation and proliferation, mediate the effects of retinoids (24).

β-carotene is an antioxidant and a potent quencher of free radicals such as the highly reactive singlet oxygen. At lower partial pressures of oxygen, associated with early transformation of normal cells, β-carotene acts as an antioxidant and peroxidation inhibitor (25, 26). At higher partial pressures of oxygen, it acts as a pro-oxidant and could become an auto-oxidizer. Once the transformation process has progressed towards completion (promotion), or is fully completed, it could inhibit cell growth, in its pro-oxidant form. It has also been shown to be an immunostimulant (22, 27).

Vitamin E is a potent antioxidant and a well known quencher of free oxygen radicals. It is an inhibitor of peroxidation at quite high oxygen pressures (25). It has been found to protect cells from carcinogenic chemicals by inhibiting lipid peroxidation and its damaging free-radical-mediated consequences (28). It also produces immuno-enhancement.

NAC, a precursor of extracellular and intracellular glutathione, is a potent antioxidant and detoxificant. It inhibits adduct formation by either ingested or inhaled carcinogens. NAC is effective at the initiation stage of carcinogenesis (29, 30). In vitro, NAC inhibits mutagens such as aflatoxin, benzpyrene and cigarette smoke condensate (31).

Naturally occurring algae such as S. fusiformis are rich in carotenoids, vitamin E and other micronutrients. Animal studies have established that it is a potent inhibitor of hamster buccal pouch carcinogenesis (32). It is likely that the micronutrients mediate its chemopreventive activity. Studies among preschool children in southern India revealed that it is a rich natural source of provitamin A which improves the serum level of retinol in vitamin A-deficient children (33). Alcohol and water extracts of Spirulina have been found to inhibit lipid peroxidation, and thus they might be effective against free-radical-induced lipid peroxidation, which in turn may lead to cellular transformation (34).

Safety of the currently used chemopreventive agents

Since chemopreventive substances are administered to apparently healthy and normal subjects, at doses considerably higher than their recommended daily allowances, and for prolonged periods, these agents should not result in severe toxic side-effects or long-term sequelae. Any toxicity, if it does occur, should be mild and acceptable; furthermore, it should be reversible when administration is

stopped. It is important to have information on the nature of toxicities encountered, for different doses and durations of administration, in order to define the dosage and duration of supplementation to be used in clinical trials aimed at establishing the chemopreventive efficacy of these agents.

Information on vitamin A toxicity can be derived from dermatological practice involving high-dose vitamin A for prolonged periods, from studies of the population consuming vitamin A supplements, including those who have consumed large doses unwittingly over prolonged periods, and from chemopreventive studies. There is a distinct possibility that there are mild toxic symptoms of vitamin A in these studies that have not been recognized. The safety and toxicity profile of retinoids, based on the above studies, have been extensively reviewed (35, 36, 37).

The clinical toxicity of vitamin A includes manifestations such as skin and mucous membrane desquamation, skin rashes, skin erythema, itching, alopecia, epistaxis, headache, nausea, vomiting, diarrhoea, insomnia, irritability, ataxia, bone pains, hepatomegaly, papilloedema and hypertriglyceridaemia. The concern about retinol-induced liver damage stemmed from a number of observations related to overconsumption of vitamin A supplements. Although there have been sporadic reports of cirrhosis appearing after many years of heavy vitamin A overadministration, there is no evidence that serious liver damage will occur if vitamin A is administered at a dose of 300 000 IU/day for up to 2 years. Mild and transient liver enzyme abnormalities occur with prolonged retinoid use. It results in elevated serum triglyceride levels, although not of the alarming magnitude observed in patients with pre-existing risk factors or hypertriglyceridaemia.

For substances like vitamin A, which tend to bio-accumulate, the chronicity of exposure and the presence of predisposing conditions such as liver diseases are crucial when considering toxicity. One review concluded that the scientific information available on vitamin A toxicity is not sufficient to identify either a specific maximum threshold intake for its adverse effects or an upper safe limit of intake (36). An intake of 10 000 IU/day cannot be guaranteed to be safe for all individuals in a large population. On the other hand, an intake of ~25 000 IU/day does not cause adverse effects in all individuals.

However, the overall evidence from many studies indicates that vitamin A is a safe supplement and may be well tolerated for long periods (37, 38). The major side-effects were limited to skin and mucous membrane desquamation and dryness during treatment. The toxic side-effects were reversed when supplementation was stopped or the dosage was reduced. A majority of patients were able to sustain a daily dose of 300 000 IU over a long supplementation period. An Italian chemopreventive study, which administered 300 000 IU/day for at least 12 months to 138 subjects with resected stage 1 lung cancers, concluded that high-dose retinyl palmitate administration was a well tolerated and safe treatment (37). In a large European chemoprevention study (EUROSCAN), it is being administered at a dose of 300 000 IU/day in the first year and 150 000 IU/day in the second year (29). A recent report from a large American study involving vitamin A (25 000 IU/day for 5 years) revealed only a negligible increase in serum triglyceride levels (39).

The level of toxicity associated with synthetic analogues such as isotretinoin was unacceptable when used at a dosage of 2 mg/kg body weight (40). More than three-quarters of the subjects had toxic side-effects, but when used at lower doses (0.5–1 mg/kg body weight) the toxicity was observed in a quarter of the subjects (41). Toxic side-effects were experienced by half of the subjects supplemented with etretinate (42) and by less than a quarter of subjects on 4-HPR (43). The toxicity profile of natural analogues of vitamin A (e.g. retinyl palmitate) appears to be more acceptable than that of synthetic analogues.

Several reviews have established that β-carotene is a safe supplement, as compared with equivalent amounts of vitamin A (44). It has been successfully used to treat inherited photosensitivity diseases for more than 15 years, at dosages of 180 mg/day or more, without any side-effects other than hypercarotenaemia. It does not cause hypervitaminosis A. The yellowing of the skin, which sometimes accompanies high intakes, disappears when the carotene ingestion is discontinued. Agents such as vitamin E and NAC have been shown to be safe supplements (29, 30, 44). The blue-green alga S. fusiformis has been used as a food item by natives of Africa and South America for many years. It has been shown to be safe in toxicological studies and studies involving children in southern India (45).

End-points evaluated in reported head and neck cancer chemoprevention trials

Head and neck cancer chemoprevention trials have evaluated the agents in terms of different end-points. Some trials have evaluated the ability of chemopreventive agents to reverse or prevent recurrence of oral leukoplakia and to maintain the response (40, 41, 43, 46, 47, 48, 49, 50, 51, 52). Other trials have used successfully treated head and neck cancer patients to evaluate whether chemopreventive agents could prevent loco-regional recurrences and second primary cancers (30, 42, 53, 54). Some studies, including a few of the above, evaluated the modulation of biomarkers of carcinogenesis, such as dysplastic changes, cytonuclear morphometry, cellular features and micronucleated cell counts (MNCs; 55, 56). No study has evaluated the primary outcome in terms of the reduction in head and neck cancer incidence and mortality rates in apparently healthy subjects.

Intermediate end-points, such as precancerous lesions, and biomarkers of carcinogenesis, such as micronuclei (MNCs), are useful for rapid evaluation of chemopreventive agents before long-term, cost-intensive phase III trials with cancer incidence as the end-point are considered. The most widely studied biomarkers in head and neck cancer chemoprevention trials are MNCs, which are intracellular fragments of extranuclear DNA, representing ongoing and recent DNA damage. Even though they provide a quantitative measure of DNA damage, they are non-specific. MNCs have not been found to be a valid intermediate biomarker in head and neck cancer chemoprevention studies (47, 57, 58). Biomarkers such as proliferating cell nuclear antigen (PCNA) and various cytokeratins are currently being evaluated as intermediate end-points. Even if many biomarkers do not prove to be effective surrogates for cancer incidence, they could help in establishing optimal agents, doses and schedules for evaluation in phase III trials and in studying compliance with chemoprevention.

Studies with retinoids

The ability of vitamin A analogues such as all trans-retinoic acid (tretinoin), etretinate, and 13-cis retinoic acid (isotretinoin or 13-cRA) to induce objective

Table 1. Early chemoprevention studies on the effect of retinoids on oral precancerous lesions[a]

Author (year)[a]	Agent	No.	Dose	Clinical response (%)	
Rysser (1971)	B-all tRA	10	20–100 mg × 4–15 months	7	(70%)
Stuttgen (1975)	B-all tRA	8	40–60 mg × 3–4 months	8	(100%)
Raque (1975)	B-all tRA	5	100 mg × 2 weeks–4 months	5	(100%)
Koch (1978)	B-all tRA	27	70 mg × 2 months	6	(59%)
	13-cRA	24	70 mg × 2 months	21	(87%)
	Etretinate	24	70 mg × 2 months	20	(83%)
Koch (1981)	Etretinate	24	50 mg + 0.1% paste × 6 weeks	20	(83%)
	Etretinate	21	75 mg × 6 weeks	15	(71%)
Cordero (1981)	Etretinate	3	1 mg/kg × 2 months–6 years	3	(100%)
Shah (1983)	13-cRA	11	3–10 mg/day × 6 months	9	(82%)

[a]Cited in Lippman, Benner & Hong (59).
No., number of subjects; tRA, transretinoic acid; 13-cRA, 13-cis retinoic acid.

clinical responses (a combination of complete and partial responses and stable disease) in oral leuko-plakias was initially observed in non-randomized studies involving systemic administration and/or topical applications of these agents (Table 1; cited in 59). However, these treatments were associated with considerable toxicity, particularly mucocutaneous toxicity, with relapses after cessation of therapy.

The results of two placebo-controlled random-ized trials of retinoids, with remission of oral leuko-plakia as the end-points, are given in Table 2. A higher proportion of complete responses (~ 55%) was reported with natural analogues of vitamin A (retinyl acetate or palmitate) in southern Indian pan tobacco chewers than was observed (~ 8%)

with 13-cRA (40, 46). Dysplasia was reversed in 13/24 (54%) subjects on 13-cRA, compared with 2/20 (10%) subjects on a placebo (40). Within 2–3 months of stopping the supplements, the lesions reappeared. The major toxic side-effects observed with 13-cRA were cheilitis, facial erythema, and dry-ness and peeling of skin in 79% (19/24), conjunc-tivitis in 54% (13/24), and hypertriglyceridaemia in 71% (17/24) of subjects. The frequency of toxic symptoms was higher in those who received a dose of 2 mg/kg than it was in those who received 1 mg/kg; 47% (8/17) of those receiving 2 mg/kg required a dose reduction because of toxicity.

In our study, a reduction in the frequency of MNCs was observed in 96% of subjects (46), although

Table 2. Results of placebo-controlled randomized trials of the effects of retinoids on oral leukoplakia

Author (year)	Agent (No.)	Dose	Response (%)		
			CR	PR	NR
Hong et al. (1986)	Isotretinoin (24)	1–2 mg/kg/day	2 (8)	14 (58)	6 (25)
	Placebo (20)	× 6 months	0 (0)	2 (10)	16 (80)
Stich et al. (1988)	Vitamin A (21)	200 000 IU/week	12 (57)	–	9 (43)
	Placebo (33)	× 6 months	1 (3)	–	32 (97)

No., number of subjects; CR, complete response; PR, partial response; NR, no response.

complete remission of leukoplakia was only observed in 57%. In the group receiving a placebo, seven new leukoplakias were observed, compared with none in the group receiving vitamin A. Histological examination of baseline biopsy specimens in subjects on vitamin A revealed a loss of polarity of basal cells in 72.2%, lymphocyte infiltration in 66.7% and nuclei with condensed chromatin in 72.2% of subjects; these features were seen in 22.2%, 5.5% and 0%, respectively, of biopsy specimens collected after completion of supplementation. No toxic side-effects were observed in this study. Four months after stopping the administration of vitamin A, the frequency of MNCs increased, and the lesions started to recur. In another study involving 61 chewers, with MNCs as the end point, the reduced frequency of MNCs induced by high-dose vitamin A treatment could be sustained for prolonged periods by low-dose (50 000 IU/week) maintenance therapy (49).

Cytomorphometry was also evaluated in our study. Nuclear textures of oral mucosal cells were examined by quantitative image analysis, using paraffin-embedded biopsies from five complete responders to vitamin A taken before, at the end of, and 4 months after treatment (60). They were stained with Feulgen reaction before undergoing quantitative image analysis of two parameters: variance of intensity and entropy. Both these parameters were significantly reduced in all five as a result of vitamin A treatment. During the post-treatment period, nuclei with condensed chromatin, as measured by the variance of intensity, reappeared in the mucosa of four of the five subjects, although no visible recurrences were observed.

Results of a randomized chemoprevention trial with fenretinide (4-HPR), in subjects surgically treated for oral leukoplakia, were reported by Chiesa et al. (43). At the time of reporting, 115 subjects had been randomized after surgical excision of leukoplakia to receive either 200 mg of fenretinide daily for 52 weeks or a placebo; 80 subjects had completed the 1-year intervention – 41 in the control group and 39 in the fenretinide arm. A quarter of the control arm had non-homogeneous lesions compared with one-third of the study group. Twelve (29%) relapses were observed in the control group compared with three (8%) in the 4-HPR group. Treatment was generally well tolerated: two subjects had skin dryness, two showed hyperbilirubinaemia, and one showed hypertriglyceridaemia.

A recently reported randomized trial by Lippman et al. (41) evaluated the efficacy of low-dose 13-cRA and β-carotene in maintaining the response induced by high-dose 13-cRA. In the first phase of the study, 70 subjects with leukoplakia underwent induction therapy with 13-cRA (1.5 mg/kg body weight) for 3 months. Following 3 months of therapy, MNC counts significantly reduced (57). However, the reduction in the frequency of micronuclei was not consistently associated with a clinical or histological response to treatment. In 59 subjects, no further progression occurred (lesions stable or regressing). In the second phase of the study, they were further randomized to receive maintenance therapy with either low-dose isotretinoin (n = 26, 0.5 mg/kg) or β-carotene (n = 33, 30 mg/day). In 23 of the 52 subjects who could be histologically evaluated – 4 with responses, 14 with stable lesions and 5 with disease progression – the clinical and histological responses

Author (year)	Agent	No.	Disease progression			Second primary	
			Local (%)	Reg. (%)	Dist. (%)	H&N (%)	Other (%)
Bolla et al. (1994)	Etretinate	156	12 (8)	7 (5)	19 (12)	12 (8)	16 (10)
	Placebo	160	11 (7)	8 (5)	10 (6)	13 (8)	16 (10)
Benner et al. (1994)	13-cRA	49	5 (10)	8 (16)	8 (16)	3[a] (6)	4 (8)
	Placebo	51	7 (14)	7 (14)	5 (10)	13[a] (25)	3 (6)

Table 3. Placebo-controlled randomized trials of vitamin A in treated head and neck cancer patients

No., number of subjects; Reg., regional lymph node relapse; Dist., distant relapse; H&N, head and neck sites; Other, other sites.
[a]Second primaries in head and neck sites as well as in lung.

Table 4. Studies of the effect of β-carotene on oral leukoplakias

Author (year)	Dose	No.	% CR	% PR	% OR
Garewal et al. (1990)[a]	30 mg/day × 3–6 months	24	8	63	71
Malaker et al. (1991)	30 mg/day × 6 months	18	–	–	44
Garewal et al. (1992)[a]	60 mg/day × 6 months	39	–	–	56
Toma et al. (1994)	90 mg/day × 9 months	23	33	11	44

No., number of subjects; CR, complete response; PR, partial response; OR, observed response.
[a]Cited in Garewal (52).

were in agreement. However, 10 of the subjects with clinical disease progression had features of stable histological disease. Ninety-two per cent of the 13-cRA group and 45% of the β-carotene group responded to maintenance treatment. The proportion of complete responses was not reported. The overall frequency of disease progression was significantly higher (55%) in the group taking β-carotene than it was in the 13-cRA group (8%). While on maintenance, *in situ* carcinoma developed in one subject in each group and invasive oral cancer developed in five subjects in the β-carotene group. Toxicity was greater with both isotretinoin induction and maintenance therapies than it was with β-carotene: during the induction phase, skin dryness was observed in 95%, cheilitis in 94%, conjunctivitis in 50% and hypertriglyceridaemia in 76% of subjects. The above features were observed in 83%, 92%, 54% and 58% of subjects, respectively, during the maintenance phase of 13-cRA, although a significant proportion were a result of low-grade toxicity. However, with respect to mucocutaneous toxicity, there were no significant differences in the proportion of high-grade (grade 3 or 4) reactions between the two treatment groups.

Table 3 shows the results of two randomized trials that evaluated the efficacy of retinoids in preventing loco-regional recurrences and second primary tumours in subjects who had their primary head and neck cancers controlled by surgery and/or radiotherapy. In the study by Bolla et al. (42), supplementation was started no later than 5 days after surgery and/or the initiation of radiotherapy: 156 subjects were randomized to receive etretinate at a dose of 50 mg/day during the first month, followed by a dose 25 mg/day during the subsequent 23 months; and 160 subjects were

randomized to receive a placebo. The 5-year survival rate and disease-free survival rate were similar in the two groups (64% in the etretinate group and 75% in the placebo group). There were no significant differences in loco-regional, distant recurrences or in the frequency of second primary tumours between the treatment groups. Toxic side-effects were observed in 51% of subjects on etretinate, compared with 26% on placebo.

The report by Benner et al. (54) updated the information from an earlier study (53) at a median follow-up of 54.5 months. A total of 49 subjects received isotretinoin at a dose of 50–100 mg/m² per day for 12 months and 51 received a placebo. There was no difference in the frequencies of recurrence of the original tumour between the isotretinoin and the placebo groups. However, there was a statistically significant reduction in the rate of development of second primary tumours in the 13-cRA arm. Isotretinoin appeared to have had a greater impact on reducing the occurrence of second primaries within the carcinogen-exposed field of upper aerodigestive tract and lungs than within the body as a whole. The proportion of subjects in the 13-cRA arm with moderate to severe toxic side-effects was as follows: skin dryness, 63%; cheilitis, 24%; hypertriglyceridaemia, 26%; and conjunctivitis, 18%. A total of 18% did not complete treatment because of toxicity.

A European trial evaluating the chemopreventive efficacy of retinyl palmitate (300 000 IU/day for 12 months) in treated stage I lung cancer patients reported a 33% reduction in the frequency of second primary cancers in the treated arm as compared with the control arm (61).

There are now major ongoing studies recruiting large numbers of treated head and neck cancer patients in order to evaluate the efficacy of vitamin A

Table 5. Placebo-controlled randomized trials of the effect of β-carotene on oral leukoplakia					
Author (year)	Dose	No.	CR (%)	PR (%)	NR (%)
Stich et al. (1988)	180 mg/week × 6 months	27	4 (15)	4 (15)	19 (70)
	Placebo	33	1 (3)	7 (21)	25 (76)

No., number of subjects; CR, complete response; PR, partial response; NR, no response.

(retinyl palmitate) and 13-cRA (30 mg/daily) in reducing recurrences and second primaries (*30, 62*).

Studies with β-carotene

β-carotene has been shown to reduce the frequency of MNCs in tobacco users (*47, 55*). The efficacy of β-carotene in reversing oral leukoplakia has been evaluated in a few single-arm studies (Table 4) and two randomized controlled trials (Table 5). The single-arm studies involved few subjects and complete responses were reported in less than one-third of them. No significant toxic side-effects were observed in these studies.

The outcome of one randomized trial is shown in Table 5. When β-carotene was used at a dose of 180 mg/week for 6 months, the complete regression of leukoplakias was observed in 4 out of 27 (15%) subjects who could be evaluated (*47*). During the trial period, four new leukoplakias occurred in the β-carotene group compared with seven in the placebo arm. The frequency of MNCs, which was elevated at baseline both in cells scraped from leukoplakia and in the normal-appearing mucosa, reduced to normal levels in 34/35 (97%) subjects after 3 months on β-carotene. In another study involving betel quid chewers with MNCs as the end-point, β-carotene

administered at 60 mg/week was less effective in maintaining the suppression of MNCs induced by high-dose β-carotene (180 mg/week; *50*).

In the maintenance study by Lippman et al. (*41*) described previously, leukoplakic lesions progressed in 16 out of 29 (55%) subjects who were randomized to receive maintenance therapy with β-carotene (30 mg/day × 9 months). Invasive or *in situ* carcinoma developed in six subjects in the β-carotene group compared with one in the retinoid group.

No reported study has addressed the potential of β-carotene to prevent loco-regional failures or second primaries in treated head and neck cancer patients. An ongoing study in the United States is evaluating the potential of β-carotene (50 mg/day) to prevent second primaries and relapses (cited in *59*).

Studies with vitamin E and other substances

Table 6 shows the outcomes of studies investigating the chemopreventive efficacy of agents other than carotenoids and retinoids. Recently a single-arm phase II trial with vitamin E has been reported (*51*). Of the 43 subjects with oral leukoplakia who were given 400 IU of vitamin E (α-tocopherol) twice daily for 24 weeks, 20 (46%) showed clinical responses and 9 (21%) showed histological responses.

Table 6. Studies of the effects of agents other than retinoids and carotenoids on oral leukoplakia						
Author (year)	Agent	Dose	No.	CR (%)	PR (%)	NR (%)
Benner et al. (1993)	Vitamin E	800 IU/day × 6 months	43	10 (23)	10 (23)	11 (26)
Toma, Palumbo & Rosso (1994)	Selenium	300 µg/day × 3 months	18	2 (11)	5 (28)	11 (61)
Mathew et al. (1995)	*Spirulina fusiformis*	1 g/day × 12 months	44	20 (45)	5 (11)	19 (44)

No., number of subjects; CR, complete response; PR, partial response; NR, no response.

Complete clinical responses were observed in 10/43 (23%), partial responses in 10/43 (23%) and stable disease in 8/43 (18%) subjects. Complete histological responses were not observed in any lesion, and partial histological responses were observed in 9/43 (21%) subjects. Response rates did not vary appreciably with the size of the lesion. Clinical responses were observed in 14/27 (52%) subjects in which the maximum dimension was 1.5 cm or more, and in 4/11 (36%) subjects in which the maximum dimension was 3 cm or more. The frequency of MNCs, which at baseline was higher in the lesion than in the normal-appearing mucosa, decreased in all subjects on vitamin E, and thus there was no significant association between the reduction in MNCs and either clinical or histological responses (58).

Selenium was evaluated for chemopreventive efficacy in a preliminary study by Toma, Palumbo & Rosso (63). Eighteen subjects with oral precancerous lesions were given 300 ug/day of selenium for 3 months. The objective response frequency was 38.8%, with two complete responses and five partial responses. The progression of lesions was observed after cessation of therapy.

The chemopreventive potential of a naturally occurring blue-green alga S. fusiformis was evaluated in a group of tobacco chewers in Kerala (64). The administration of 1 g of Spirulina daily for 1 year resulted in complete regression of leukoplakias in 20 out of 44 (45%) subjects; the response was more pronounced in small lesions and homogeneous lesions. The lesions recurred in 9/20 complete responders within 1 year of the supplementation of Spirulina. Malignant transformation of the lesion was observed in two subjects on Spirulina. No major toxic side-effects were observed during or after administration.

A major study in Europe is currently evaluating the potential of N-acetylcysteine, either alone or in combination with vitamin A, to prevent relapses and second primaries in previously treated head and neck cancer patients. The results are awaited (29).

Studies with combination of micronutrients

Muñoz et al. (56) did not observe a reduction in the frequency of MNCs in buccal mucosal epithelial cells in a double-blind intervention trial of the effect of riboflavin (200 mg/week), retinol (50 000 IU/week) and zinc (50 mg/week) among 200 Chinese subjects.

Stich et al. (47) reported on a study in which 51 betel quid chewers with oral leukoplakias were supplemented with 180 mg/week of β-carotene plus 100 000 IU/week of vitamin A for 6 months. The frequency of MNCs was greatly reduced both in samples from leukoplakia (4.01 ± 1.05 at baseline versus 1.16 ± 0.94) and in samples from the normal-looking mucosa (4.18 ± 0.78 versus 1.22 ± 0.88). Complete regression of the lesions was observed in 14/51 (28%), partial regression in 4/51 (7%) and no response in 33/51 (65%) subjects. Four new lesions developed among subjects on supplement. No toxic side-effects were observed as a result of supplementation.

An ongoing study in the United States is evaluating a combination of 30 mg β-carotene daily plus 25 000 IU vitamin A daily in subjects with oral leukoplakia (59).

A large European study (EUROSCAN) is evaluating the efficacy of a combination of retinyl palmitate and NAC in reducing the occurrence of second primary tumours in treated head and neck cancer patients (30).

Methods of monitoring compliance

Compliance with drug dosage and regime is important for the proper evaluation of the efficacy and toxicity of chemopreventive agents. In our early studies (46, 47), compliance was ensured by a nurse administering the supplements to the participants. In our later studies, the pill intake was monitored by a nurse who counted the leftover pills at monthly refills. Larger intervention studies have relied on monitoring pill intake by pill counts (30). Serial measurements of blood concentration of micronutrients or their metabolites and the modulation of biomarkers of carcinogenesis such as MNCs, in either all the participants or a sample of them, are also useful in determining the compliance. Chemopreventive trials have established that the prolonged administration of β-carotene and vitamin E results in an elevation of serum levels of these compounds (51, 65, 66). The prolonged administration of vitamin A results in an elevation of the mean peak level of the esterified fraction of retinol in the serum (67, 68).

Micronutrient interactions

The evaluation of potential interactions of administered micronutrients, both with each other and with other micronutrients, is important for designing future studies. In a short-term phase I toxicity trial of supplemental β-carotene in normal volunteers, Xu et al. (*69*) reported a progressive decrease in the serum concentration of α-tocopherol during 9 months of daily supplementation. Another study, involving a small number of postoperative colon cancer patients supplemented with β-carotene for 3 months, reported a significant decrease in the serum concentration of α-tocopherol (*70*). This was disturbing in the context of reports that suggested an inverse relationship between the incidence of both cancer and coronary artery disease and serum α-tocopherol concentration. However, observations from several other studies found no evidence of a decreased concentration of α-tocopherol in subjects supplemented with either long-term β-carotene or vitamin A (*66, 71*). Similarly, supplementation with vitamin A, vitamin E and vitamin C does not seem to alter serum levels of β-carotene (*66, 72*).

Conclusions

Consistent observations have been reported from chemopreventive studies of head and neck cancer conducted in different regions of the world. The studies in Western countries have involved head and neck carcinogenesis associated with cigarette smoking and alcohol drinking, while the studies in India involved lesions caused by the complex mixture of betel quid chewing with or without bidi/cigarette smoking and/or alcohol drinking. A significant proportion of oral leukoplakias regressed following supplementation, but in the long run the lesions reappeared once the supplements were stopped. Supplementation did not affect the occurrence of loco-regional recurrences in treated head and neck cancer patients; however, a reduction in the frequency of second primaries was observed with 13-cRA (*54*) but not with etretinate (*42*). Large studies with both natural and synthetic analogues of vitamin A are ongoing in order to evaluate this aspect further.

There are no data available that demonstrate a reduction in the incidence and mortality rates of oral and other head and neck cancers as a result of using this approach, although lower frequencies of malignant transformations were observed in a small number of leukoplakic subjects receiving retinoids (*41*) compared with subjects receiving β-carotene.

Although retinoids seem to have a significant activity in head and neck carcinogenesis, compared with β-carotene (*41, 46, 47*), there is considerable toxicity associated with the administration of synthetic analogues of retinoids (*40, 41*). Further studies are required to evaluate the chemopreventive activity of vitamin E in head and neck cancer.

No intermediate biomarkers have yet been validated for cancer incidence. A panel of biomarkers such as PCNA, cytokeratins and others are being evaluated. MNCs have not proved to be a valid surrogate intermediate biomarker, but they may be useful in monitoring the compliance of subjects.

In summary, retinoids and β-carotene have been shown to result in the regression of oral leukoplakia, but the lesions recur soon after stopping the administration of chemopreventive agents. Retinoids seem to be more effective than carotenoids in reversing oral leukoplakias. Whether prolonged administration of retinoids could result in a reduction in head and neck cancer incidence and mortality rates is not known, and trials are required in this direction. It is also important to identify and evaluate other potential and less toxic chemopreventive agents. Any attempt at chemoprevention of head and neck cancer should be undertaken within the framework of experimental studies only. At present, it is premature to suggest chemoprevention as a routine strategy to prevent head and neck cancer.

References

1 Parkin DM, Pisani P, Ferlay J. Estimates of the worldwide incidence of eighteen major cancers in 1985. *Int J Cancer*, 1993, 54:594–606.

2 Pisani P, Parkin DM, Ferlay J. Estimates of the worldwide mortality from eighteen major cancers in 1985: implications for prevention and projections of future burden. *Int J Cancer*, 1993, 55:891–903.

3 Jayant K, Yeole BB. Cancers of the upper alimentary and respiratory tracts in Bombay, India: a study of incidence over two decades. *Br J Cancer*, 1987, 56:847–852.

4 Zaidi SHM. Cancer trends in Pakistan. In: Khogali M et al., eds. *Cancer Prevention in Developing Countries*. Oxford, Pergamon Press, 1986:69–73.

5 Coleman MP et al. *Trends in Cancer Incidence and Mortality*. IARC Scientific Publications No.121. Lyon, International Agency for Research on Cancer, 1993.

6 de Flora S et al. Prevention of induced lung tumours in mice by dietary N-Acetylcysteine. *Cancer Lett*, 1986, 32:235–241.

7 Shklar G, Schwartz J. Oral cancer inhibition by micronutrients. The experimental basis for clinical trials. *Oral Oncol, Eur J Cancer*, 1993, 29:9–16.

8 Graham S et al. Dietary factors in the epidemiology of cancer of the larynx. *Am J Epidemiol*, 1981, 113:675–680.

9 Marshall J et al. Diet in the epidemiology of oral cancer. *Nutr Cancer*, 1982, 3:145–149.

10 Ziegler RG. A review of epidemiologic evidence that carotenoids reduce the risk of cancer. *J Nutr*, 1989, 119:116–122.

11 Steinmetz KA, Potter JD. Vegetables, fruit, and cancer. I. Epidemiology. *Cancer Causes Control*, 1991, 2:325–357.

12 Barone J et al. Vitamin supplement use and risk of oral and esophageal cancer. *Nutr Cancer*, 1992, 18:31–41.

13 Block G, Patterson B, Subar A. Fruit, vegetables and cancer prevention: a review of the epidemiological evidence. *Nutr Cancer*, 1992, 18:1–29.

14 Gridley G et al. Vitamin supplement use and reduced risk of oral and pharyngeal cancer. *Am J Epidemiol*, 1992, 135:1083–1092.

15 Slaughter DP, Southwick HW, Smejkel W. 'Field cancerization' in oral stratified squamous epithelium: clinical implications of multicentric origin. *Cancer*, 1953, 6:963–968.

16 Tepperman BS, Fitzpatrick PJ. Second respiratory and upper digestive tract cancers after oral cancer. *Lancet*, 1981, ii:547–549.

17 Haughey BH et al. Meta-analysis of second malignant tumours in head and neck cancer: the case for an endoscopic screening protocol. *Ann Otol Rhinol Laryngol*, 1992, 101:105–112.

18 Day GL, Blot WJ. Second primary tumours in patients with oral cancer. *Cancer*, 1992, 70:14–19.

19 Day GL et al. Second cancers following oral and pharyngeal cancer: patients' characteristics and survival patterns. *Oral Oncol, Eur J Cancer*, 1994, 30:381–386.

20 Lotan R, Dennert G. Stimulatory effects of vitamin A analogues on induction of cell mediated cytotoxicity *in vivo. Cancer Res*, 1979, 39:55–58.

21 Spern M, Roberts A. Role of retinoids in differentiation and carcinogenesis. *J Natl Cancer Inst*, 1984, 73:1381–1387.

22 Prabhala RH et al. The effects of 13-cis-retinoic acid and beta-carotene on cellular immunity in humans. *Cancer*, 1991, 67:1556–1560.

23 Smith SA et al. Retinoids in cancer therapy. *J Clin Oncol*, 1992, 10:839–864.

24 Goss GD, McBurney MW. Physiological and clinical aspects of vitamin A and its metabolites. *Critical Rev Clin Lab Sci*, 1992, 29:185–215.

25 Burton GW, Ingold KV. B-carotene: an unusual type of lipid antioxidant. *Science*, 1984, 224:569–573.

26 Palozza P, Krinski NI. Beta carotene and alpha tocopherol are synergistic antioxidants. *Arch Biochem Biophys*, 1992, 297:184–187.

27 Schwartz JL, Flynn E, Shklar G. The effect of carotenoids on the antitumour immune response *in vivo* and *in vitro* with hamster and mouse immune effectors. *Ann NY Acad Sci*, 1990, 587:92–109.

28 Borek C. Vitamin E as an anticarcinogen. *Ann NY Acad Sci*, 1990, 570:417–420.

29 de Vries N, van Zandwijk N, Pastorino U. Chemoprevention in the management of oral cancer: EUROSCAN and other studies. *Oral Oncol, Eur J Cancer*, 1992, 28:153–157.

30 de Vries N, Pastorino U, van Zandwijk N. Chemoprevention of second primary tumours in head and neck cancer in Europe: EUROSCAN. *Oral Oncol Eur J Cancer*, 1994, 30:367–368.

31 de Flora S, Bennicelli C, Zanacchi P. *In vitro* effects of N-acetylcysteine on the mutagenecity of direct acting compounds and procarcinogens. *Carcinogenesis*, 1984, 5:505–510.

32 Schwartz J, Shklar G. Regression of experimental hamster cancer by beta carotene and algae extracts. *J Oral Maxillofac Surg*, 1987, 45:510–515.

33 Annapurna V et al. Bioavailability of Spirulina carotenes in preschool children. *J Clin Biochem Nutr*, 1991, 10:145–151.

34 Manoj G, Venkatraman, LV, Srinivas L. Antioxidant properties of Spirulina extracts. In: Seshadri CV, Jeegi Bai N, eds. *Spirulina Ecology, Taxonomy, Technology, Applications National Symposium*. Madras, MCRC, 1992:148–154.

35 Bendich A, Langseth L. Safety of vitamin A. *Am J Clin Nutr*, 1989, 49:358–371.

36 Hathcock N et al. Evaluation of vitamin A toxicity. *Am J Clin Nutr*, 1990, 52:183–202.

37 Pastorino U et al. Safety of high-dose vitamin A. *Oncology*, 1991, 48:131–137.

38 Omenn GS et al. The B-carotene and retinol efficacy trial (CARET) for chemoprevention of lung cancer in high risk populations: smokers and asbestos-exposed workers. *Cancer Res*, 1994, 54, 2038s–2043s.

39 Omenn GS et al. Long term vitamin A does not produce clinically significant hypertriglyceridemia: results from CARET, the B-carotene and retinol efficacy trial. *Cancer Epidemiol Biomark Prev,* 1994, 3:711–713.

40 Hong WK et al. 13-cis-retinoic acid in the treatment of oral leukoplakia. *N Engl J Med,* 1986, 315:1501–1505.

41 Lippman SM et al. Comparison of low dose isotretinoin with beta carotene to prevent oral carcinogenesis. *N Engl J Med,* 1993, 328:15–20.

42 Bolla M et al. Prevention of second primary tumours with etretinate in squamous cell carcinoma of the oral cavity and propharynx. Results of a multicentric double blind randomised study. *Eur J Cancer,* 1994, 30:767–772.

43 Chiesa F et al. Prevention of local relapses and new localisations of oral leucoplakias with the synthetic retinoid Fenretinide (4-HPR). Preliminary results. *Oral Oncol, Eur J Cancer,* 1992, 28:97–102.

44 Bendich A. The safety of B-carotene. *Nutr Cancer,* 1988, 11:207–214.

45 Seshadri CV, Jeeji Bai N, eds. *Spirulina Ecology, Taxonomy, Technology, Applications National Symposium.* Madras, MCRC, 1992.

46 Stich HF et al. Response of oral leukoplakias to the administration of vitamin A. *Cancer Lett,* 1988, 40:93–101.

47 Stich HF et al. Remission of oral leucoplakias and micronuclei in tobacco/betel quid chewers treated with beta-carotene and with beta-carotene plus vitamin A. *Int J Cancer,* 1988, 42:195–199.

48 Malaker K et al. Management of oral mucosal dysplasia with B-carotene retinoic acid: a pilot cross over study. *Cancer Detect Prev,* 1991, 15:335–340.

49 Stich HF et al. Remission of precancerous lesions in the oral cavity of tobacco chewers and maintenance of the protective effect of B-carotene or vitamin A. *Am J Clin Nutr,* 1991, 53:298s–304s.

50 Stich HF et al. Remission of oral precancerous lesions of tobacco/arecanut chewers following administration of B-carotene or vitamin A, and maintenance of the protective effect. *Cancer Detect Prev,* 1991, 15:93–98.

51 Benner SE et al. Regression of oral leukoplakia with alpha-tocopherol: a community clinical oncology program chemoprevention study. *J Natl Cancer Inst,* 1993, 85:44–47.

52 Garewal HS. Beta-carotene and vitamin E in oral cancer prevention. *J Cell Biochem,* 1993, 17:262–269.

53 Hong WK et al. Prevention of second primary tumours with isotretinoin in squamous-cell carcinoma of the head and neck. *N Engl J Med,* 1990, 323:795–801.

54 Benner SE et al. Prevention of second primary tumours with isotretinoin in patients with squamous cell carcinoma of the head and neck: long term follow up. *J Natl Cancer Inst,* 1994, 86:140–41.

55 Stich HF, Hornby AP, Dunn BP. A pilot beta-carotene intervention trial with Inuits using smokeless tobacco. *Int J Cancer,* 1985, 36:321–327.

56 Muñoz N et al. Effect of riboflavin, retinol, and zinc on micronuclei of buccal mucosa and of oesophagus: a randomized double-blind intervention study in China. *J Natl Cancer Inst,* 1987, 79:687–691.

57 Benner SE et al. Micronuclei, a biomarker for chemoprevention trials: results of a randomized study in oral pre-malignancy. *Int J Cancer,* 1994, 59:457–459.

58 Benner SE et al. Reduction in oral mucosa micronuclei frequency following alpha-tocopherol treatment of oral leukoplakia. *Cancer Epidemiol Biomark Prev,* 1994, 3:73–76.

59 Lippman SM, Benner SE, Hong WK. Retinoids in chemoprevention of head and neck carcinogenesis. *Prev Med,* 1993, 22:693–700.

60 Stich HF et al. Quantitation of chromatin patterns by image analysis as a predictive tool in chemopreventive trials with vitamin A. In:Vainio H, Sorsa M, McMicheal AJ, eds. *Complex Mixtures and Cancer Risk.* IARC Scientific Publication No. 104. Lyon, International Agency for Research on Cancer, 1990:151–163.

61 Pastorino U, Infante M, Maiola M. Adjuvant treatment of stage I lung cancer with high-dose vitamin A. *J Clin Oncol,* 1993, 11, 1216–1222.

62 Lippman SM, Benner SE, Hong WK. Retinoid chemoprevention studies in upper aerodigestive tract and lung carcinogenesis. *Cancer Res,* 1994, 54:205s–208s.

63 Toma S, Palumbo R, Rosso R. Results, toxicity and compliance in chemoprevention trials of head and neck cancer. *Eur J Cancer Prev,* 1994, 3:63–68.

64 Mathew B et al. Evaluation of chemoprevention of oral cancer with *Spirulina fusiformis. Nutr Cancer,* 1995, 24:197–202.

65 Albanes D et al. Serum B-carotene before and after B-carotene supplementation. *Eur J Clin Nutr,* 1992, 46:15–24.

66 Nierenberg DW et al. Steady-state serum concentration of alpha tocopherol not altered by supplementation with oral beta carotene. *J Natl Cancer Inst*, 1994, 86:117–120.

67 Alberts DS et al. Pharmacokinetics and metabolism of retinol administered at a chemopreventive level to normal subjects. *Cancer Detect Prev*, 1988, 13:55–64.

68 Plezia PM et al. The role of serum and tissue pharmacology studies in the design and interpretation of chemoprevention trials. *Prev Med*, 1989, 18:680–687.

69 Xu MJ et al. Reduction in plasma or skin alpha-tocopherol concentration with long term administration of B-carotene in humans and mice. *J Natl Cancer Inst*, 1992, 84:1559–1565.

70 Mobarhan S et al. B-carotene supplementation results in an increased serum and colonic mucosal concentration of B-carotene and a decrease in alpha-tocopherol concentration in patients with colonic neoplasia. *Cancer Epidemiol Biomark Prev*, 1994, 3:501–505.

71 Goodman GE, Metch BJ, Omenn GS. The effects of long-term B-carotene and vitamin A administration on serum concentrations of alpha-tocopherol. *Cancer Epidemiol Biomar Prev*, 1994, 3:429–32.

72 Willett WC et al. Vitamins A, E, and carotene: effects of supplementation on their plasma levels. *Am J Clin Nutr*, 1983, 38:559–566.

R. Sankaranarayanan
Unit of Descriptive Epidemiology, International Agency for Research on Cancer, 150 cours Albert Thomas, 69372 Lyon cedex 08, France

B. Mathew, C. Varghese, R. Jyothirmayi and M. Krishnan Nair
Regional Cancer Centre, Trivandrum, Pin 695011, Kerala, India

P.P. Nair
Human Nutrition Research Centre, Bldg 308, 10300, Baltimore Avenue, Beltsville, MD 20705, USA

T. Somanathan,
Department of Pathology, Armed Forces Medical College, Pune - 40, India

Chemoprevention of oesophageal cancer

N. Muñoz* and E. Buiatti

The most recent estimates of the worldwide incidence of oesophageal cancer (mainly squamous cell carcinoma) rank it ninth among the most frequent cancers, with about 300 000 new cases per year, but it ranks sixth among cancer deaths because of its high fatality rate (1, 2). Its descriptive epidemiology is strongly dominated by a variability (related to geography, gender and ethnicity) in incidence and mortality rates and other trends. Male:female incidence ratios indicate that, while in Europe and America men are more exposed to risk factors than women, in the very high-risk populations of Asia, the exposure tends to be similar in both sexes. This heterogeneous pattern strongly suggests a multifactorial environmental aetiology, with alcohol and tobacco having a greater role in America and Europe, while nutritional and other factors are more involved in the high-risk areas of central Asia and China.

Several case–control studies in Western countries have illustrated the important roles of tobacco and alcohol, which appear to act according to a multiplicative model. Some of these studies have also shown a clearly independent effect of each of these factors (3). In Western Europe and North America, 90% or more of the risk of oesophageal cancer can be attributed to alcohol and tobacco smoking. In central Asia, China and other high-risk developing countries, however, these two risk factors appear to be of negligible importance. Opium smoking, chewing of opium pipe scrapings, tobacco and other chewings, ingestion of pickled vegetables, and the habit of drinking hot beverages such as *maté* have been identified as relevant risk factors in some of these populations. However, in both types of oesophageal cancer, i.e. both related and unrelated to alcohol and tobacco, a monotonous diet that is poor in fresh fruits and vegetables, and therefore deficient in vitamins and other micronutrients, has been a common denominator (4). This finding is in accordance with the very high risk of oesophageal cancer in Plummer-Vinson syndrome, which is associated with iron and vitamin deficiencies.

*Correspondence: N. Munõz, Unit of Field and Intervention Studies, International Agency for Research on Cancer, 150 cours Albert Thomas, 69372 Lyon cedex 08, France.

Dietary deficiencies, acting through micronutrient-dependent enzyme systems, might alter the rate of activation or deactivation of precarcinogens and thus accelerate early or late stages of carcinogenesis. This point is of crucial relevance when estimates are made of the possible impact of intervention with dietary supplements to prevent these effects, in which the timing and dose of the dietary supplement are under question (4).

Various histological lesions of the oesophageal mucosa have been proposed as possible precancerous lesions. They include chronic oesophagitis, atrophy and dysplasia (5). The correlation between their prevalence and the risk of oesophageal cancer in various populations, their age distribution, their location in the oesophagus, and their progression and regression rates in follow-up studies are all in accordance with their being precancerous (6, 7). These lesions could be a potential target for secondary prevention programmes, but their cytological diagnostic criteria are not unequivocal, as indicated by the low predictive value of the abrasive cytology as a screening test (4). This might explain the rather disappointing impact of cytological screening in reducing mortality for oesophageal cancer in China (4), thus pointing out the crucial relevance of primary prevention programmes for decreasing the risk of this highly lethal cancer.

Primary prevention efforts have been directed at reducing the consumption of alcohol and tobacco, and supplementing the diet with micronutrients. While some progress has been achieved in the control of alcohol and tobacco in Western countries, tobacco consumption is rising by 1–2% each year in developing countries (3).

Several published and ongoing trials deal with the possible preventive effect of nutritional supplements in relation to oesophageal cancer; some have as end-points the neoplasia itself, and others use early end-points such as precancerous lesions. These trials are summarized in Table 1. All are being conducted in populations that are at high risk of oesophageal cancer.

The Huixian trial

Surveys in the populations at high risk of oesophageal cancer in Henan Province, China, revealed

Table 1. Study design and results of published intervention trials on oesophageal cancer

Authors, area	Subjects	No.	Study design	Treatment	Dose	Follow-up	End-points	Results
Published trials								
Muñoz et al. (4), Wahrendorf et al. (11) China, Huixian County	Random population sample, 35–64 years	610	Double-blind, placebo control	Retinol Riboflavin Zinc	15 mg/week 200 mg/week 50 mg/week	13.5 months	Prevalence of oesophageal lesions; prevalence of micronuclei in oesophageal mucosa	No effect
Blot et al. (13) China, Linxian County	General population in three communes, 40–69 years	29 584	Factorial	A: retinol + zinc B: riboflavin + niacin C: vitamin C + molybdenum D: β-carotene + vitamin E + selenium		5 years	Incidence and mortality	No effect
Li et al. (15) China, Linxian County	Severe oesophageal dysplasia	3318	Double-blind, placebo control	Multivitamin/ multimineral factor		5 years	Incidence and mortality	No effect
Zaridze et al. (16) Uzbekistan	Men, 55–69 years, with chronic oesophagitis	300	2 × 2 factorial	Riboflavin Vitamin A + carotene + vitamin E	200 mg/week 30 mg/week 280 mg/week 40 mg/week	20 months	Changes in precancerous lesions	Non-significant effect of β-carotene, retinol and vitamin E
Wang (18) China	With hyperplasia or dysplasia, 25–75 years	254	Randomized, placebo control	Calcium	600 mg/day	7 months	Profile of epithelia proliferating cells	No effect
Han (19) Linxian, China	Oesophageal dysplasia	1705	Randomized, placebo control	Retinoid, herbs		5 years	Incidence of cancer	43% reduction in incidence

Table 1. (contd) Study design and results of published intervention trials on oesophageal cancer

Authors, area	Subjects	No.	Study design	Treatment	Dose	Follow-up	End-points	Results
Ongoing trials								
Qiu China, Huixian County	With oesophagitis + hyperplasia and/or dysplasia	200	Double-blind placebo control	Calcium	1200 mg/day	1 year	Changes in precancerous lesions	
Yang China, Huixian County	With chronic oesophagitis; with hyperplasia and/or dysplasia	600	Randomized	200 subjects – calcium 400 subjects – herb R	1200 mg/day		Incidence and mortality	

that blood levels of various micronutrients, particularly riboflavin, were consistently low (8). These observations motivated this trial.

The results of this study, which is the first controlled nutritional intervention study in cancer epidemiology, have been published elsewhere (9, 10, 11) and can be summarized as follows.

The aim of this randomized double-blind intervention trial was to determine whether a combined treatment with retinol, riboflavin and zinc could result, after 1 year, in a lower prevalence of precancerous lesions of the oesophagus among the group receiving the active treatment as compared with the group receiving a placebo. A random sample of 610 subjects, aged 35–64 years, was drawn from two production brigades. These subjects were randomly split into two groups of 305 each. One group received the active treatment (15 mg [50 000 IU] retinol, 200 mg riboflavin and 50 mg of zinc) once a week, and the other group received a placebo, which consisted of identical-looking capsules administered weekly. The capsules were distributed by 'barefoot doctors'.

The study subjects were interviewed, underwent a physical examination and had blood samples taken both at entry into the study and at the end of the treatment, 13.5 months later.

Compliance with the treatment, as assessed by inspection of follow-up records kept by the 'barefoot doctors' and by changes in the blood levels 2 and 13.5 months after beginning treatment, was excellent. The final examination of the 567 subjects (93%) also included oesophagoscopy, with at least two biopsies taken. Histological slides were read independently and blindly by three pathologists. After a final diagnosis was reached by consensus, the code for treatment assignment was opened. The prevalence of micronuclei was also evaluated. For these studies, smears were prepared from exfoliated cells obtained from the buccal mucosa and oesophagus of subsamples of 200 and 170 subjects, respectively.

Two end-points were used to evaluate the effect of the treatment: the prevalence of precancerous lesions and the prevalence of micronucleated cells in the oesophageal mucosa.

The prevalence of oesophagitis, with or without atrophy or dysplasia, was 45.3% in the placebo group and 48.9% in the vitamin-treated group. Oesophagitis was accompanied by atrophy in 12.7% and dysplasia in 2.2% in the placebo group, and by atrophy in 12.3% and dysplasia in 2.5% in the vitamin-treated group. Although no reduction in the prevalence of histologically diagnosed precancerous lesions was observed, a significantly lower prevalence of oesophageal micronucleated cells was found in the group receiving a combined treatment of riboflavin, retinol and zinc over 13.5 months (0.19%), as compared with the control group (0.31%, $P = 0.04$; 9, 10). The reduction of oesophageal micronucleated cells could represent an effect of treatment at an early stage of the carcinogenesis process. One difficulty in the final interpretation of this trial arises from the fact that, at the end of the trial, an increase in blood retinol levels occurred in 47% of subjects in the placebo group and in 76% of those receiving the treatment. The corresponding figures for riboflavin were 17% and 66%. These changes in blood levels of the vitamins were probably the result of dietary changes that occurred during the study period (12). To account for these changes a multivariate analysis was carried out.

The results showed a reduction in the prevalence of precancerous lesions in those whose blood levels of retinol, riboflavin and zinc improved or remained unchanged, as compared with those whose levels got worse during the study period (11).

The overall results of this trial suggest a beneficial effect of retinol, riboflavin and zinc on the prevalence of precancerous lesions, but they also illustrate the difficulty of evaluating intervention trials using nutrient supplementation in populations in which rapid changes in dietary habits are occurring. This is happening in China as a consequence of changes in economic policy, which are resulting in a higher and wider availability of foods.

The Linxian trials

Two large-scale intervention studies have been conducted in the same high-risk population in China, in which a subclinical deficiency of several micronutrients was identified.

General population trial

A total of 29 584 adults, aged 40–69 years, were randomized according to a 2^4 factorial design into one of eight vitamin/mineral supplement combinations. The factorial design allowed the assessment of four nutrient combinations: retinol + zinc; riboflavin + niacin; ascorbic acid + molybdenum; and β-carotene + selenium + α-tocopherol. Doses ranged

from 1–2 times US Recommended Daily Allowances. Cancer incidence and mortality were ascertained during March 1986 and May 1991 and were used as end-points.

Mortality among trial participants was ascertained via follow-up by village doctors. Diagnoses of cancer were ascertained via local commune and county hospitals, and supplemented by a study medical team that provided clinical and diagnostic services, including endoscopy, for participants with symptoms suggestive of oesophageal or stomach cancer.

Statistical analyses focused on estimating the effects of supplementation with each of the four vitamin/mineral factors during a 5.25-year period (March 1986 – May 1991) on total mortality and cancer mortality rates. Incidence and mortality rates were calculated for oesophageal, gastric cardia, other stomach and other cancers. Proportional hazard regression analyses were employed to estimate relative risks of mortality and cancer incidence, and corresponding 95% confidence intervals for the four main effects after adjustment for matching variables.

A total of 2127 deaths occurred among trial participants during the intervention period. Cancer was the leading cause of death, with 32% of all deaths being due to oesophageal or stomach cancer, followed by cerebrovascular disease (25%). Significantly ($P = 0.03$) lower total mortality (RR = 0.91; 95% CI = 0.84–0.99) occurred among those receiving supplementation with β-carotene, vitamin E and selenium. The reduction was mainly due to lower cancer rates (RR = 0.87; 95% CI = 0.75–1.00), especially stomach cancer (RR = 0.79; 95% CI = 0.64–0.99), with the reduced risk beginning to arise about 1–2 years after the start of supplementation with these vitamins and minerals. A non-significant reduction in oesophageal cancer mortality was observed in those receiving β-carotene + vitamin E + selenium (RR = 0.96), retinol + zinc (RR = 0.93) and riboflavin + niacin (RR = 0.90).

Patterns of cancer incidence, on the basis of 1298 cases, generally resembled those for cancer mortality. Oesophageal cancer incidence was lower in those receiving riboflavin and niacin (RR = 0.86, 95% CI = 0.74–1.01), but no significant changes occurred in the other treatment groups. The apparent lack of effect of vitamin C in this trial deserves further discussion.

In this trial, the difference in the plasma vitamin levels between the treatment and control groups was much smaller than expected: during the intervention, plasma vitamin C levels rose from 0.15 to 0.81 mg/dl in the treatment group and from 0.25 to 0.54 mg/dl in the control group. This indicates that, in the presence of a considerable increase in the intake of most of the vitamins being evaluated in the trial, because of the changes in economic policy mentioned above, there was substantial contamination of the control group, and this considerably reduced the power of the study to detect effects of these micronutrients (13).

In a subset of 391 individuals from the two villages involved in the main trial, an endoscopy was performed at the end of intervention in order to evaluate the effect of treatment on the prevalence of early invasive cancer and dysplasia of the oesophagus and stomach. Fifteen per cent of the subjects had early cancer or dysplasia, but no differences were seen between treatment and placebo groups, except for a non-significant reduction of gastric neoplasias in the group that received retinol + zinc (14).

Oesophageal dysplasia trial

A second trial was conducted among 3318 people with a cytological diagnosis of oesophageal dysplasia; these subjects were derived from the same population as the previous trial. They were randomly assigned to receive a daily supplementation for 6 years of either 14 vitamins and 12 minerals or a placebo. Doses were 2–3 times US Recommended Daily Allowances. This design is not informative with regard to the effect of individual nutrients.

Compliance was assessed by counting unused pills monthly for all trial participants and by assaying nutrient levels in blood collected from samples of individuals randomly selected without replacement every 3 months throughout the trial. Cancers were identified through routine surveillance and by special cytology and endoscopy screenings after 2.5 years and 6 years.

Mortality and incidence rates of oesophageal/gastric cardia cancer during the 6-year intervention period were compared between those receiving vitamin/mineral supplements and those receiving a placebo. The relative risks for end-points were estimated using Cox proportional hazard and logistic regression models.

After the follow-up at the end of 6 years, 128 cases of oesophageal cancer were identified in the placebo group (cumulative incidence rate 7.7%) and 123

cases in the supplement group (cumulative incidence rate 7.4%; RR = 0.94; 95% CI = 0.73–1.20).

Cumulative oesophageal death rates were 16% lower (RR = 0.84; 95% CI = 0.54–1.29) among individuals receiving supplements than among those receiving the placebo, a difference that was not significant ($P > 0.10$; 15).

Monitoring of blood levels of vitamins during the 6-year intervention showed clear increases in retinol, riboflavin, ascorbic acid and β-carotene in the treatment group, while only a slight increase in riboflavin was observed in the placebo group. Thus, the lack of effect cannot be ascribed to contamination of the placebo group as in the previous trial.

In summary, this trial did not show any effect of mineral/vitamin supplements on the incidence or mortality rates of oesophageal cancer (15).

Other trials

Another trial based on nutritional supplementation has been initiated in an area in Uzbekistan where there is a high risk of oesophageal cancer. A total of 300 males with a histological diagnosis of chronic oesophagitis were randomized into one of four groups, receiving treatment with retinol (100 000 IU), α-tocopherol (40 ml), β-carotene (280 mg) and riboflavin (200 mg) or placebo, according to a 2 × 2 factorial design. Using progression-regression rates of precancerous lesions as endpoints, preliminary results after 20 months of treatment suggest possible protective effects for β-carotene and for a high α-tocopherol/cholesterol ratio, but the difference was not significant (16).

Two randomized trials on the effect of calcium supplementation on oesophageal precancerous lesions are ongoing in China (17, 18). The study subjects are males from a high-risk area and with a diagnosis of oesophagitis. Totals of 200 and 600 subjects have been randomized into groups receiving treatment with either calcium (1200 mg/day) or placebo in one trial and groups receiving either calcium (1200 mg/day), herb R or placebo in the other trial. A published paper on one of the trials reports some preliminary results showing no significant effect of calcium supplementation compared with the placebo group (18).

Finally, a synthetic retinoid [N-4 (ethoxycarbophenyl) retinamide] and traditional chinese medicine has also been used in a trial involving over 1700 subjects with oesophageal dysplasia in

Linxian, China. After a 5-year follow-up, a reduction in the incidence of oesophageal cancer was reported in the group receiving the retinoid and the group receiving Chinese traditional medicine, as compared with the placebo group (*19*).

Conclusion

A monotonous diet poor in fresh vegetables and fruits has been the common denominator for both types of oesophageal cancer, i.e. those strongly associated with alcohol and tobacco and those unrelated to these two factors. Thus, it has been postulated that the decreasing trends in oesophageal cancer mortality in some European countries, and the moderate increase in others, despite increases in the consumption of tobacco and alcohol, might be due to the protection afforded by the increasing intake of fruits (*19*).

A diet that is low in fresh vegetables and fruits results in a low intake of carotenes and vitamin C, which are known to be necessary to maintain the integrity of the oesophageal mucosa. In addition, observational epidemiological studies have shown that a higher intake or blood level of antioxidant vitamins is associated with a lower risk of oesophageal cancer.

To test the hypothesis that the protective effect of a diet rich in fresh vegetables and fruits is mediated through β-carotene, vitamin C and other micronutrients, randomized trials have been conducted in high-risk populations in China and Uzbekistan. These trials have not shown a clear protective effect for precancerous lesions or oesophageal cancer.

There are various possibilities that might explain these negative or inconclusive results:

- The concurrent dietary changes taking place in China during the intervention period resulted in a substantial contamination of the control or placebo group and reduced considerably the power of the various trials to detect an effect.
- The doses used and the treatment and follow-up periods were not sufficient to detect an effect of the various micronutrients.
- In those trials using precancerous lesions as an end-point, an additional difficulty is the possibility of misclassification of the various lesions because of a lack of clear diagnostic criteria.
- Fruits and vegetables exert a protective effect by mechanisms that do not involve β-carotene, vitamin C or the other micronutrients tested.

References

1 Parkin DM, Pisani P, Ferlay J. Estimates of the worldwide incidence of eighteen major cancers in 1985. *Int J Cancer*, 1993, 54:594–606.

2 Pisani P, Parkin DM, Ferlay J., Estimates of worldwide mortality from eighteen major cancers in 1985: implications for prevention and projections of future burden, *Int J Cancer*, 1993, 55:891–903.

3 Muñoz N, Castellsagué X, Epidemiology of oesophageal cancer, *Eur J gastroenterol Hepatol*, 1994, 6:649-655.

4 Muñoz N, Day NE, Oesophagus. In: Schottenfeld D, Fraumeni JF, Jr, eds. *Cancer Epidemiology and Prevention*, 2nd ed. In press.

5 Muñoz N et al. Precursor lesions of esophageal cancer in high-risk populations in Iran and china. *Lancet*, 1982, i:876–879.

6 Crespi M et al. Precursor lesions of oesophageal cancer in a low-risk population in China: comparison with high-risk populations. *Int J Cancer*, 1984, 34:599-602.

7 Dawsey SM et al. Esophageal cytology and subsequent risk of esophageal cancer. A prospective follow-up study from Linxian, China. *Acta Cytol*, 1994, 38:183–192.

8 Thurnham DI et al. Comparison of riboflavin, vitamin A and zinc status in high- and low-risk regions for oesophageal cancer in China. *Nutr Cancer*, 1985, 7:131–143.

9 Muñoz N et al. No effect of riboflavine, retinol and zinc on the prevalence of precancerous lesions of the esophagus. A randomized double-blind intervention study in a high-risk popualation in China. *Lancet*, 1985, ii:111–114.

10 Muñoz N et al. Effect of riboflavin, retinol and zinc on micronuclei of buccal mucosa and of oesophagus: a randomzied double-blind intervention study in China. *J Natl Cancer Inst*, 1987, 79:687–691.

11 Wahrendorf J et al. Blood, retinol and zinc riboflavin status in relation to precancerous lesions of the esophagus: findings from a vitamin intervention trial in the People's Republic of China. *Cancer Res*, 1988, 48:2280–2283.

12 Thurnham DI et al. Nutritional and haematological status of Chinese farmers: the influence of 13.5 months treatment with riboflavin, retinol and zinc. *Eur J Clin Nutr*, 1988, 42:647–660.

13 Blot WJ et al. Nutrition intervention trials in Linxian, China: Supplementation with specific vitamin/mineral combinations, cancer incidence, and disease-specific mortality in the general population. *J Natl Cancer Inst*, 1993, 85:1483–1492.

14 Wang GQ et al. Effects of vitamin/mineral supplementation on the prevalence of histological dysplasia and early cancer of the esophagus and stomach: results from the general population trial in Linxian, China. *Cancer Epid Biomarkers Prev*, 1994, 3:161–166.

15 Li JY et al. Nutritional intervention trials in Linxian, China: multiple vitamin/mineral supplementation, cancer incidence, and disease-specific mortality among adults with esophageal dysplasia. *J Natl Cancer Inst*, 1993, 85:1492–1498.

16 Zaridze D, Evstifeeva T, Boyle P. Chemoprevention of oral leukoplakia and chronic esophagitis in an area of high incidence of oral and esophageal cancer. *Ann Epidemiol*, 1993, 3:225–234.

17 Coleman M., Wahrendorf J, eds. *Directory of On-going Research in Cancer Epidemiology*. IARC Sci. Publ. No. 110. Lyon, International Agency for Research on Cancer, 1992.

18 Wang LD. Effect of added dietary calcium on human esophageal precancerous lesions in a high risk area for esophageal cancer – A randomized double-blind intervention trial. *Chung Hua Chung Liu Tsa Chih* [English summary], 1990, 12:332–335.

19 Han J. Highlights of the cancer chemoprevention studies in China. *Prev Med*, 1993 22:712–722.

N. Muñoz
Unit of Field and Intervention Studies,
International Agency for Research on Cancer,
150 cours Albert Thomas, 69372 Lyon cedex 08 France

E. Buiatti
Epidemiology Unit, Centre for Cancer Study and
Prevention, Florence, Italy

Chemoprevention of stomach cancer

E. Buiatti* and N. Muñoz

Although rates of gastric cancer (GC) have been decreasing in most populations, it still remains the second most common cancer worldwide (1), with an estimated 755 000 new cases per year. The absolute number of new cases per year is not decreasing, mainly because of the ageing of Western populations in which most of the decreasing mortality trends are seen, suggesting that the impact of GC on public health will still be very high in the future.

Substantial epidemiological evidence is available from many case–control and some cohort studies on the determinants of GC risk; briefly, these are represented by a monotonous diet that is poor in fresh fruits and vegetables and in which salt and preserved foods are highly represented (2, 3), and by the active infection with *Helicobacter pylori*, a bacteria adapted to the gastric environment (4). The most consistent observational epidemiology data refer to the protective effect of a diet that is high in fruit and fresh vegetables, and this has been confirmed in studies involving a wide range of populations with a wide dietary variability. In several of these studies, the estimated intakes or the serum levels of β-carotene, vitamin C and, to a lesser extent, α-tocopherol were also inversely related to GC risk; the carotenoids and ascorbic acid were mainly derived from fruits and vegetables, while the α-tocopherol sources varied in the different populations.

These findings illustrate the potential preventive effect of a balanced diet with a high proportion of fresh foods, and strongly suggest a possible role for micronutrients, such as carotenoids, ascorbic acid and α-tocopherol, as preventive agents for GC, either through their antioxidant action at a local level or by general diffusion through the bloodstream and secondary secretion into the gastric lumen. An anticarcinogenic effect of antioxidants is clearly shown in many experimental studies (5). A possible relationship between *H. pylori* infection and ascorbic acid levels in the stomach is also under investigation, as some studies point out that, in the presence of *H. pylori* infection, ascorbic acid is low in the stomach, independently of whether it comes from the dietary or supplementary intake, suggesting that

the effect of *H. pylori* could be at least partially mediated through its effect on antioxidants (6).

Strong evidence indicates that in the intestinal type of GC a series of lesions of the gastric mucosa, which behave as precancerous lesions, precede the occurrence of GC. These are chronic atrophic gastritis (CAG), with or without intestinal metaplasia (IM), and dysplasia (Dys), representing a continuum of changes from normal mucosa to carcinoma, the complete process taking at least two decades (7). In some studies, but not all, dietary factors identified as inversely or positively associated with GC were also found to be associated with these precancerous lesions (8, 9).

Recent population-based survival data show that, even in Western countries, 5-year relative survival rates for GC are very low (around 20%) and improvement over time is small (10). In the absence of widely available and effective screening programmes, primary prevention by decreasing exposure to the identified risk factors for the disease or by increasing protection against them might be the most effective way of controlling it.

Intervention trials based on chemoprevention

Despite the fact that most of the epidemiological evidence on GC concerns diet, no intervention trial on diet and stomach cancer is in progress and none is planned.

The main reasons for this are the logistical difficulties associated with changing the diet at a population level, especially in developing countries, and the tendency towards changes in the same direction in the placebo group as in the treatment group. This latter tendency occurs mainly in Western countries in which a substantial proportion of the population takes vitamin supplements, and in developing countries that are undergoing rapid economic change, such as China, which is influencing the food supply.

Two chemoprevention trials are in progress in high-risk areas, while a third one is planned in low/intermediate-risk areas in Europe. The main features of these trials are summarized in Table 1.

Chemoprevention trial in Venezuela

This trial has been running since 1992 in an area in Venezuela where there is a high risk of GC,

*Correspondence: E. Buiatti, Epidemiology Unit, Centre for Cancer Study and Prevention, Florence, Italy.

Table 1. Study design of ongoing intervention trials on gastric cancer

Authors, area	Subjects	No.	Study design	Treatment	Dose	Follow-up	End-points
Correa, Colombia	CAG[b], IM[c] + dysplasia	700	Double-blind, placebo control, factorial 2×2	Phase I: anti-H. pylori × 2 weeks; Phase II: β-carotene / vitamin C	25 mg/day / 2 g/day	3 years	Changes in precancerous lesions
Muñoz, Venezuela	GC, CAG, IM, dysplasia	2200	Double-blind, placebo control	Vitamin C + β-carotene + vitamin E	750 mg/day / 18 mg/day / 600 mg/day	3 years	Changes in precancerous lesions
Reed, ECP–IM[a], Europe	IM	1200	Double-blind, placebo control	Phase I: anti-H. pylori; Phase II: vitamin C	2 g/day	3 years	Changes in precancerous lesions

[a] European Cancer Prevention – Intestinal Metaplasia Study Group.
[b] Chronic atrophic gastritis.
[c] Intestinal metaplasia.

and an early detection programme for GC based on double-contrast X-ray and endoscopy is ongoing (11).

A total of 2200 subjects permanently resident in the State of Tachira, Venezuela, have been randomized into treatment and placebo groups. The subjects, aged 35–69 years and in general good health, were called for a gastroscopic examination after abnormalities at X-ray and agreed to participate in the trial. Treatment consists of three capsules per day for 3 years of a combination of ascorbic acid (250 mg), α-tocopherol (200 mg) and β-carotene (6 mg) or a placebo. At baseline, the following are performed: a gastroscopy with seven biopsies (two frozen, five used for histological examination), a physical examination, and blood sampling for determination of micronutrients. A simplified dietary questionnaire is also filled out. At 12, 24 and 36 months after the start of the trial, a physical examination and blood sampling are undertaken. Endoscopy is repeated at 36 months, except for IM type III and dysplasia cases, who are at high risk of GC (12) and are therefore examined every 6 months. Compliance is assessed by counting the capsules left in the bottles and will be validated by monitoring of micronutrient plasmatic levels.

The outcomes of the trial are the progression and regression rates of precancerous lesions in the treated group as compared with the placebo group. A power estimation, based on baseline progression/regression rates measured in a similar population in Colombia (7), indicates that this study should have an 80% power to detect a 50% reduction in the net progression of gastric precancerous lesions.

In the planning phase of the study, the combination of antioxidant treatment with treatment for H. pylori eradication in a factorial design was considered, since in this population adults show a prevalence of active *H. pylori* infection as high as 94%. The results of two pilot randomized trials aimed at evaluating the eradication rates using two different anti-*H. pylori* treatment strategies showed that in this population only a very low eradication rate can be achieved, possibly because of antibiotic-resistant *H. pylori* strains or high reinfection rates (*13*). Therefore the final trial design does not include *H. pylori* eradication.

Preliminary results are available from several baseline studies on the participating subjects and from a case–control study conducted on the Tachira population. The prevalence of precancerous lesions is high and comparable with other high-risk populations (CAG = 48%; IM = 34%; Dys = 5%). On the other hand, micronutrient levels are comparable with those of medium-risk populations in Europe (ascorbic acid = 9 mg/l; α-carotene = 146 ug/l; β-carotene = 247 ug/l; lycopene = 158 ug/l; α-tocopherol/cholesterol = 6.9; γ-tocopherol/cholesterol = 0.3). It should be noted, however, that this plasmatic measure reflects the present and not the past level of micronutrients, the latter possibly being related to gastric cancer risk. Preliminary results from the case–control study confirm the strong protective effect of fresh vegetables and fruits, and identify as risk factors salted fish and, in particular, corn meal, which is a staple food in Venezuela (N. Muñoz, unpublished).

The Colombia chemoprevention trial

A total of 700 subjects with a histological diagnosis of CAG or IM from a high-risk area in Colombia were enrolled in this trial in 1991–92. Treatment is with ascorbic acid, β-carotene or placebo. As the *H. pylori* infection rate is very high in this population, all the *H. pylori*-positive individuals were treated for 2 weeks with a triple therapy treatment (3 × 500 mg/day amoxicillin + 4 × 260 mg/day bismuth + 750 mg/day metronidazole). Four months after treatment, 40% eradication was achieved; this allowed the randomization of *H. pylori*-positive and *H. pylori*-negative subjects into four groups, to be treated with ascorbic acid (2 g/day), β-carotene (25 mg/day), ascorbic acid + β-carotene or placebo. These are now being examined after 36 months of treatment in order to determine the progression/regression rates of gastric lesions (P. Correa, personal communication).

The European chemoprevention trial

The aim of this trial, which will involve several European populations, is to investigate the effect of ascorbic acid supplementation and *H. pylori* eradication on the rate of histological change of gastric precancerous lesions (*14*).

A total of 1200 patients of European descent, aged 20–70 years and with histologically determined IM, will first be classified according to *H. pylori* status. If found to be *H. pylori*-positive, they will be enrolled in an eradication trial; if negative, they will immediately be randomized to receive either ascorbic acid treatment or a placebo. In the eradication trial, *H. pylori*-positive subjects (expected to be 80–95%) will be randomized into treatment and placebo groups in the ratio 2:1. They will then be further randomized into the ascorbic acid treatment/placebo trial according to the success of the eradication, as assessed using the ^{13}C urea breath test 4–6 weeks after the end of treatment for *H. pylori*. Compliance will be monitored at 3-monthly intervals by tablet count, at which time eventual adverse effects will also be monitored. Ascorbic acid will be given for 3 years at a dose of 2 g/day.

This trial has been designed to test the following hypotheses:

- *Helicobacter pylori* eradication increases the regression rate and/or decreases the progression rate of IM;
- ascorbic acid supplements (2 g/day for 3 years) increase the regression rate and/or decrease the progression rate of IM.

The trial will also investigate interactions between the above-mentioned treatments.

Other studies

In China, two trials aimed at evaluating the effect of micronutrient supplementation on cancer sites other than the stomach have reported contradictory results in relation to GC.

The Linxian chemoprevention trial (*15*) on oesophageal cancer (2^4 factorial design) resulted in a non-significant reduction in GC incidence and mortality rate (non-cardia GCs) in the group treated with selenium + β-carotene + vitamin E (RR = 0.82, 95% CI = 0.56–1.20 for incidence, and RR = 0.72, 95% CI = 0.46–1.14 for mortality). When GCs as a whole were considered, the relative risks reached borderline significance. In a subset of 391 subjects from the same trial on whom an endoscopy was performed to evaluate the prevalence of oesophageal and gastric precancerous and cancerous lesions, the results from the group treated with retinol + zinc suggested a possible protective effect of this treatment against GC (RR = 0.38, 95% CI = 0.13–1.15, $P = 0.088$), while no effect was seen in the group treated with selenium + β-carotene + vitamin E (16). In addition, in the second trial involving 3318 subjects with prior cytological evidence of oesophageal dysplasia, an increase in both the incidence and mortality rate of non-cardia gastric cancer was observed in the group receiving a combination of 14 vitamins and 12 minerals (including β-carotene, vitamin E and selenium) as compared with those receiving a placebo [RR (incidence) = 3.54, 95% CI = 1.17–10.76; RR (mortality) = 2.68, 95% CI = 0.71–10.11; see 17].

In the Finland chemoprevention trial on lung cancer (18), in which 29 133 males, all heavy smokers, were treated with α-tocopherol, β-carotene, α-tocopherol + β-carotene or a placebo, 70 incident cases of GC appeared in both treatment groups against 56 in the placebo group (the difference is not significant).

It should be noted, however, that the three trials are not comparable, because of differences in the baseline risks of GC (much higher in China, mainly due to gastric cardia cancers), the baseline levels of micronutrients (higher in Finland), treatment doses (somewhat higher in Finland) and treatment strategies (different combinations of micronutrients).

Concluding remarks

Stomach cancer still represents an important public health problem in many areas of the world, and primary prevention seems to be the most feasible strategy for decreasing its occurrence.

The main hypothesis underlying the three ongoing trials is that subjects at high risk of developing GC as a result of being affected by precancerous lesions could be protected by treatment with antioxidants (and by *H. pylori* eradication in two out of three trials), since, according to experimental and observational studies, antioxidants appear to prevent the progression of the lesions towards GC. The possible interaction between antioxidants and *H. pylori* infection is still not well established, and represents a research area for the future. The effects of the combined anti-*H. pylori* treatment and antioxidant supplementation are also difficult to quantify. Differences in the forthcoming results from the Venezuelan and Colombia intervention studies could possibly be due to the fact that *H. pylori* treatment is being used in the Colombian trial but not in the Venezuelan trial, as these trials are otherwise quite similar. All ongoing trials foresee the progression/regression rate of precancerous lesions as an end-point, while none of them will allow the effect of treatment on the occurrence of cancer to be evaluated unless the follow-up period is extended for many years.

None of the trials considers dietary changes as a possible preventive action. In the planning phase of the Venezuela study, this strategy was considered but then withdrawn because of its lack of feasibility in a developing country (N. Muñoz, unpublished).

Results from three trials in which the main outcomes were other cancer sites (oesophagus and lung) produced some information on the effect of dietary supplementation on GC risk, but the suggested effects are contradictory. Unexpectedly, the stomach was the one cancer site that appeared to be protected in the oesophageal cancer trial, in the group receiving treatment with β-carotene, vitamin E and selenium, but this was not confirmed in the oesophageal dysplasia trial in the same population, nor in the lung cancer trial in Finland. The result observed in the oesophageal cancer trial could be due to chance, as a result of the multiple comparisons made in this complex factorial design (the chance that one comparison could turn out to be significant at the $P < 0.03$ level was 0.11; see 15). On the other hand, the lack of an effect in the lung cancer trial could be due to the high baseline levels of nutrients in this population, the high supplement doses, or the low power of this study, which was not planned for evaluating GC as an outcome. Results from the ongoing trials might increase our understanding of the value of micronutrients in the prevention of gastric cancer.

Summary

A varied and balanced diet that is rich in fresh fruit and vegetables and poor in preserved foods is thought to represent the main protection against gastric cancer. *Helicobacter pylori* infection also appears to have a role in the disease; its eradication therefore represents another promising potential preventive measure. The effect of diet is supposed to be mediated by micronutrients with an antioxidant role, such as ascorbic acid, β-carotene and α-tocopherol, which could act on different phases of the carcinogenic process, interrupting the progression of precancerous lesions towards cancer. The two trials ongoing in Latin America and the one planned in Europe all deal with the effect of antioxidants, with or without *H. pylori* eradication, on the progression/regression rate of precancerous lesions of the stomach. The trial in Venezuela has an 80% power to detect a 50% reduction in the net progression of precancerous lesions in the group (from a high-risk population) undergoing a complex antioxidant treatment for 3 years. In this population a case–control study confirmed the protective effect of fresh fruits and vegetables in relation to gastric cancer.

Other trials, which aimed to evaluate the chemopreventive potential of micronutrients on other cancer sites, have reported contradictory results concerning gastric cancer risk. When interpreting these results the following should be considered: a possible interaction between *H. pylori* infection and the antioxidants; the baseline levels of antioxidants in these populations; and the doses and duration of treatment.

References

1 Parkin DM, Pisani P, Ferlay J. Estimates of the worldwide incidence of eighteen major cancers in 1985. *Int J Cancer*, 1993, 54:594–606.

2 Tomatis L et al. *Cancer: causes, occurrence and control.* Lyon, International Agency for Research on Cancer, 1990, (IARC Sci. Publ. No. 100).

3 Risch HA et al. Dietary factors and the incidence of cancer of the stomach. *Am J Epidemiol*, 1985, 122: 947–957.

4 Muñoz N. Is *Helicobacter pylori* a cause of gastric cancer? An appraisal of the seroepidemiological evidence. *Cancer Epid Biom Prev*, 1994, 3:445–451.

5 Gey KF, Brubacher GB, Stähelin HB. Plasma levels of antioxidant vitamins in relation to ischemic heart disease and cancer. *Am J Clin Nutr*, 1987, 45:1368–1377.

6 Sobala GM et al. Effect of eradication of *Helicobacter pylori* on gastric juice ascorbic acid concentrations. *Gut*, 1993, 34:1038–1041.

7 Correa P et al. The gastric precancerous process in a high risk population: Cohort follow-up. *Cancer Res*, 1990, 50:4737–4740.

8 Fontham E et al. Diet and chronic atrophic gastritis: a case–control study. *J Natl Cancer Inst*, 1986, 76:621–627.

9 Haenszel W et al. Serum micronutrients levels in relation to gastric pathology. *Int J Cancer*, 1985, 36:43–48.

10 National Cancer Institute. *Cancer statistics review 1973–1988.* NIH Publication no. 91-2789. Department of Health and Human Services, Bethesda, MD, 1991.

11 Buiatti E, Balzi D, Barchielli A. *Intervention trials of cancer prevention: results and new research programmes.* Lyon, International Agency for Research on Cancer, 1994. IARC Technical Report No. 18.

12 Filipe MI, Jass JR. Intestinal metaplasia sub-types and cancer risk. In: Filipe MI, Jass JR, eds. *Gastric carcinoma.* Edinburgh, Churchill Livingstone, 1986:97–115.

13 Buiatti E et al. Difficulty in eradicating *Helicobacter pylori* in a population at high risk for stomach cancer in Venezuela. *Cancer Causes Control*, 1994 5:249–254.

14 Reed PI, Johnston BJ. Primary prevention of gastric precancerous lesions. *Eur J Cancer*, 1993, 2:79–82.

15 Blot WJ et al. Nutrition intervention trials in Linxian, China: supplementation with specific vitamin/mineral combinations, cancer incidence, and disease-specific mortality in the general population. *J Natl Cancer Inst*, 1993, 85:1483–1491.

16 Wang GQ et al. Effects of vitamin/mineral supplementation on the prevalence of histological dysplasia and early cancer of the esophagus and stomach: results from the general population trial in Linxian, China. *Cancer Epidemiol Biomarkers Prev*, 1994, 3:161–166.

17 Li JY et al. Nutritional intervention trials in Linxian, China: multiple vitamin/mineral supplementation, cancer incidence, and disease-specific mortality among adults with esophageal dysplasia. *J Natl Cancer Inst*, 1993, 85:1492–1498.

18 The Alpha-Tocopherol, Beta-Carotene Cancer Prevention Study Group. The effect of Vitamin E and Beta Carotene on the incidence of lung cancer and other cancers in male smokers. *N Engl J Med*, 1994, 330:1029–1035.

E. Buiatti
Epidemiology Unit, Centre for Cancer Study and Prevention, Florence, Italy

N. Muñoz
Unit of Field and Intervention Studies, International Agency for Research on Cancer, 150 cours Albert Thomas, 69372 Lyon cedex 08, France

Chemoprevention of primary liver cancer

E. Buiatti

Primary liver cancer, which manifests mainly as hepatocarcinomas (HCCs), ranks eighth in incidence among cancer sites worldwide. The total estimated number is approximately 250 000 new cases per year (1). The ratio of incidence between low-risk and high-risk areas is 1:50. In fact, this highly lethal cancer represents a priority health problem in sub-Saharan Africa, east Asia, Southeast Asia and Melanesia. More than 90% of incident HCCs are related to environmental exposures. Of these, the main ones are HBV chronic active hepatitis with identifiable HBV surface antigen (HBsAg carrier status), HCV infection, exposure to aflatoxins through food contamination and high alcohol consumption, the latter occurring mainly in Western countries. In developing countries, the interaction between aflatoxin exposure and HBV hepatitis is thought to account for a large majority of HCC cases, and the two exposures are potentially preventable (2).

Rationale for HCC prevention based on HBV vaccination

In high-risk areas, the proportion of HCCs that are attributable to HBV is between 50 and 64% in case–control studies, and the figure is even higher in cohort studies (1).

At present, 47 countries are known to have immunization policies that include hepatitis B vaccination. In general, a reduction in the prevalence of HBsAg carriers has been shown in vaccinated children (3).

However, no information is currently available on the effect of vaccination on the incidence of HCC. Further information is also required on the long-term immunity of the vaccinated subjects and on the relevance of viral mutants. A trial on HBV vaccination and prevention of HCC that is ongoing in The Gambia is expected to contribute valuable information on these topics (4, 5, 6, 7).

Rationale for HCC prevention based on reduction of exposure to aflatoxins

The evidence of hepatic carcinogenesis due to aflatoxin B1 is based on experimental carcinogenicity studies, on molecular analysis of HCC which implicates aflatoxin in the induction of specific mutations in the p53 suppressor gene, and on ecological studies

(1). A case–control study nested in a Shanghai male cohort gives RR = 5.7 (CI = 1.3–26.0) for subjects with aflatoxin B1-DNA adducts measurable in their urine, and RR = 59.4 (CI = 16.6–212.0) for aflatoxin-positive/HBsAg-positive subjects (8). Estimates on the HCC risk attributable to aflatoxin exposure alone or associated with HBV are still uncertain; the above results, as well as others, suggest that they could both be relevant independent determinants of HCC and act as cofactors in HBV carcinogenesis (8).

Two strategies to reduce the risk from aflatoxins are now under investigation. The first is represented by programmes aimed at reducing food contamination. This may be achieved through a rapid post-harvest drying and a controlled storage of crops (9, 10, 11). The second strategy is based on potential chemopreventive factors such as Oltipraz.

Rationale for HCC chemoprevention
Oltipraz as a chemopreventive agent

Oltipraz (5-(2-pyrazinyl)-4 methyl-1,2 dithiole-3-thione) is a widely used single-dose antischistosomal drug that affects the metabolism of aflatoxin B1 in rats by inducing glutathione S-transferase, an enzyme involved in detoxification (12). Furthermore, Oltipraz given with food reduces aflatoxin-DNA adducts in rat liver by 60–90%, possibly reducing the aflatoxin-8,9-epoxide availability for DNA binding (9). The development of aflatoxin-induced hepatocarcinomas in rats is also inhibited at reasonably low doses (0.075% Oltipraz in the diet of rats treated with 25 ug aflatoxin B1 *per os* for 2 weeks gave a protection of 100%; see 13).

These characteristics, together with the results from ongoing phase 1 and 2 trials aimed at identifying safe doses and metabolic pathways during chronic administration, make Oltipraz a possible chemopreventive agent in populations exposed to aflatoxins.

A chemoprevention trial using Oltipraz is reported to be in the planning phase in a population that is highly exposed to aflatoxins in China (9; C. Wild, personal communication, 1994). In this area, HCC is frequent, and aflatoxins are a common contaminant of food supplies (14).

In this randomized trial with Oltipraz, aflatoxin-DNA adducts will be measured, with the aim of evaluating the rationale for the use of this product in populations in which a full-scale intervention in food storage is precluded by cost.

Trials of nutritional supplementation and traditional drugs

The subjects involved in these ongoing trials in China (Quidong and Guangxi) are at high risk of HCC because of the extent of their exposure to aflatoxins and HBV, because they are HBV carriers, or because other members of their family are primary liver cancer cases. The supplementation is with either selenium or green tea and herbs (*radix salvia mitiorhizae*). The rationale is based on experimental studies conducted in China, showing that selenium salts (organic and inorganic) and green tea have an inhibitory effect on aflatoxin B1-induced hepatomas in rats, and that the same effect is also produced in ducks by selenium salts (*15, 16*). Furthermore, levels of selenium in the blood in this population have been identified as being lower than those in populations at low risk of HCC (*17*). Green and black tea are under evaluation for their possible chemopreventive action, which could be linked to the phenolic compounds contained therein (*18*).

The administration of selenium supplements (5 ppm of sodium selenite/day for 5 years in a community of 20 847 people) has been associated with lower HCC incidence rates compared with those of other communities with a similar baseline incidence. (Baseline incidence in both populations: 419 per 100 000; at the end of treatment, 30.8 per 100 000 in the treated population, approximately 50 per 100 000 in the control population). At the moment, no information about compliance with treatment, age adjustment of rates, significance tests or comparability of cancer registration is available (*17*).

In one controlled trial, 226 HBsAg carriers were randomized to receive selenium (200 ug/day; selenized yeast) or a placebo for 4 years. Five HCCs developed in the placebo group during the 4 years, compared with none in the treatment group (*17*).

In another trial, 2474 subjects whose family members had developed primary liver cancer were randomized to receive treatment with selenium salts (200 ug/day) or placebo for 2 years. After this period, 1.26% of the placebo group and 0.69% of the treatment group had developed HCC (*17*).

Finally, in an ongoing trial, 3000 subjects, either HBV carriers or people who have been exposed to aflatoxins in the Guangxi province, have been randomized into three groups to receive green tea, traditional herbs or placebo. The end-point is HCC incidence. The follow-up time is not specified, and results are not available at present (*16*).

Conclusions

In principle, primary prevention of liver cancer, a relevant public health issue in many countries, is possible on the basis of its well known aetiologic factors. The most promising strategy is thought to be anti-HBV vaccination which is also expected to have a strong positive impact on chronic liver diseases, cirrhosis and general mortality. Further work is now ongoing on aflatoxin B1 exposure, and some data suggest that intervention on this exposure together with anti-HBV vaccination would significantly increase the preventive effect of the vaccination itself.

However, the requirement of a lengthy intervention with its associated high cost may partially restrict the use of hepatitis B vaccines in areas in which there is a high incidence of liver cancer. Similarly, rapid post-harvest drying of crops and controlled storage may be difficult to achieve systematically in all countries. Chemoprevention may therefore represent an additional, not an alternative, strategy for reducing HCC risk, with the aim of reducing the carcinogenic potential (and also the hepatotoxic effect) of aflatoxins in exposed individuals.

There is a suggestion that selenium supplements, in deficient populations, and green tea may have an anticarcinogenic potential, but results are not yet sufficient to confirm this. Again, a strategy based on these agents should not be an alternative, and interventions should aim to reduce the risk from the two main exposures associated with HCC.

Acknowledgement

I thank Dr C. Wild, IARC, Lyon, for his kind revision of this text.

References

1 Tomatis L et al. *Cancer: causes, occurrence and control.* International Agency for Research on Cancer, Lyon, 1990. (IARC Sci. Publ. No. 100).

2 Harris CC. Solving the viral-chemical puzzle of human liver carcinogenesis. *Cancer Epid Biomarkers Prev,* 1994, 3:1–2.

3 Chen D-S. From Hepatitis to Hepatoma: lessons from type B Viral Hepatitis. *Science*, 1993, 262:369–370.

4 The Gambia Hepatitis Study Group. The Gambia Hepatitis Intervention Study. *Cancer Res*, 1987; 47:5782–5787.

5 Ryder RW et al. Persistent Hepatitis B Virus infection and hepatoma in The Gambia, West Africa. *Am J Epidemiol*, 1992, 136:1122–1131.

6 Karthegisu VD et al. A novel hepatitis B variant in the sera of immunized children. *J Gen Virol*, in press.

7 Wild CP et al. Aflatoxin, liver enzymes and hepatitis B virus infection in Gambian children. *Cancer Epid Biomarkers Prev*, 1993, 2:555–561.

8 Qian GS et al. A follow-up study of urinary markers of aflatoxin exposure and liver cancer risk in Shanghai, People's Republic of China. *Cancer Epid Biomarkers Prev*, 1994, 3:3–10.

9 Kensler TW, Davis EF, Bolton MG. Strategies for chemoprevention against aflatoxin-induced liver cancer. In: Eaton DL, Groopman JD, eds. *The toxicology of aflatoxins*. New York, Academic Press, 1993:281–306.

10 Bosch FX, Muñoz N. Epidemiology of hepatocellular carcinoma. In: Bannasch P, Keppler D, Weber G, eds. *Liver Cell Carcinoma*. Lancaster, Kluwer Academic Publishers, 1989:3–15.

11 Peers F et al. Aflatoxin exposure, hepatitis B virus infection and liver cancer in Swaziland. *Int J Cancer*, 1987, 39:545–553.

12 Kensler TW et al. Mechanism of protection against aflatoxin tumorigenicityin rats fed 5-(2-pyrazinyl)-4-methyl-1,2-dithiol-3-thione (Oltipraz) and related 1,2-dithiol-3-thione and 1,2-dithiol-3-ones. *Cancer Res*, 1987, 47:4271–4277.

13 Roebuck BD et al. Protection against aflatoxin B1-induced hepatocarcinogenesisin F344 rats by 5-(2-pyrazinyl)-4-methyl-1,2-dithiole-3-thione (Oltipraz), predictive role of short-term molecular dosimetry. *Cancer Res*, 1991, 51:5501–5506.

14 Zhu YR, Chen JG, Huang XY. Hepatocellular carcinoma in Quidong County. In: Tang ZY, ed. *Primary liver cancer*. Berlin, China Academic Publishers, Springer-Verlag, 1989:204–222.

15 Han R-J. Studies on cancer chemoprevention in China. In: *Proceedings of the 4th International Conference on Prevention of Human Cancer, Nutrition and Chemoprevention Controversies*. AZ, University of Arizona, Tucson, 1992.

16 Liu QF. Randomized trial of Green Tea and Herbs in Prevention of Primary Hepatocellular Carcinoma in High Risk areas. In: Coleman M, Wahrendorf J, eds. *Directory of Ongoing Research in Cancer Epidemiology*. 1992, International Agency for Research on Cancer, Lyon, 1991. (IARC Sci. Publ. No. 110).

17 Yu S-Y et al. A preliminary report on the intervention trials of primary liver cancer in high-risk populations with nutritional supplementation of selenium in China. *Biol Trace Element Res*, 1991, 29:289–294.

18 Meeting report. Current strategies of cancer chemoprevention: 13th Sapporo Cancer Seminar. *Cancer Res*, 1994, 54:3315–3318.

E. Buiatti
Epidemiology Unit, Centre for Cancer Study and Prevention, Florence, Italy

European intervention trials of colorectal cancer prevention

J. Faivre*, B. Hofstad, L. Bonelli, P. Rooney and C. Couillault

Epidemiological studies have emphasized the major role played by diet in the aetiology of large bowel cancer. Attempts to identify causative or protective factors in analytical, epidemiological and experimental studies have led to some discrepancies. The time has come to test the most important hypotheses within the framework of intervention studies in order to evaluate the possibilities of primary prevention. The end-point of intervention studies cannot be invasive cancer itself. As there is considerable evidence that a high proportion of colorectal cancers arise in adenomas, adenoma recurrence and adenoma growth appear to be two of the most appropriate end-points. Two chemopreventive studies have been completed and three are ongoing in Europe. They all evaluate the effect of the intervention on adenoma recurrence, and the Oslo study additionally considers the effect on adenoma growth. Oral supplementation with calcium (1.5–2 g/day) is evaluated in three studies (in combination with vitamins and antioxidants in one study), vitamins and antioxidants in two studies, dietary fibre (ispaghula husk) in one study and lactulose in one study. The Modena study suggests that vitamins (A, C and E), and to a lesser extent lactulose, have a protective effect on adenoma recurrence. The low compliance (only 25% of subjects had a colonoscopy after 2 years) limits the conclusions of this study. A small study in Nottingham did not find any protective effect of calcium on adenoma recurrence. The results of ongoing studies will be available within 2–3 years. If one of the evaluated interventions proves efficient, the benefits of a simple, safe and inexpensive prophylactic for a very common cancer will be clear.

Introduction

It has recently been shown that colorectal cancer is the most common cancer in the European Community, with an estimated 135 000 new cases each year (1). With a 30% 5-year survival rate in

*Correspondence: J. Faivre, Registre des Tumeurs digestives (Equipe associée INSERM-DGS), Faculté de Médecine, 7 Boulevard Jeanne d'Arc, 21033 Dijon cedex, France

population-based statistics, its prognosis remains poor (2). Faced with this situation, it seems most likely that primary or secondary prevention will be required to control the disease. Many epidemiological studies have emphasized the major role of diet in the aetiology of colorectal cancer. Attempts to identify causative or protective factors in case–control studies or cohort studies have led to certain discrepancies (3). It is important to test the most valuable hypotheses within the framework of intervention studies in order to evaluate the possibilities of a primary prevention. The objective of this report is to review study designs and available results from randomized colorectal cancer chemoprevention trials carried out in Europe. This review does not include studies with non-specific intermediate biomarkers such as mucosal proliferation changes.

Population under study

Five complementary chemopreventive studies are being, or have already been, conducted in Europe. (Table 1) The results of one trial, the Modena study, have been published, and four trials are ongoing: studies in Oslo, Genova and Nottingham and a multicentred study proposed by the Colon Group of the European Cancer Prevention Organization (ECP).

All five European studies include patients with at least one adenoma, i.e. subjects affected by a precancerous lesion (4, 5, 6, 7, 8). The reason for this is that there is considerable evidence that a high proportion of colorectal cancers arise in adenomas. Several arguments maintain that the adenoma-carcinoma sequence is a multistep process. According to this hypothesis, factors causing the development of an adenoma *per se* should differ from those influencing the growth of a small adenoma and those influencing malignant change in a large adenoma. Colorectal cancer can be prevented by intervening at any of these stages. The aim of the four European studies is to test the effectiveness of chosen supplements on the new formation rate of adenomas. The Oslo study also has the additional aim of evaluating the effect of the intervention on the growth rate of an adenoma less than 1 cm in diameter left *in situ* in the large bowel.

Study (reference)	Main end-point	Chemopreventive agents	Number of randomized subjects	Duration of the intervention (years)
Modena (4)	Adenoma recurrence	• Vitamins A (30 000 IU) + E (20 mg) + C (1 g) • Lactulose (20 g) • No treatment	209	1–3
Oslo (6)	Adenoma growth	• Calcium (1.6 g) + β-carotene (15 mg) + vitamin E (75 mg) + vitamin C (150 mg) + selenium (101 mg) • Placebo	116	3
European Cancer Prevention Organization (ECP)(5)	Adenoma recurrence	• Calcium (2 g) • Ispaghula husk (3.8 g) • Placebo	663	3
Nottingham (7)	Adenoma recurrence	• Calcium (1.5 g) • Placebo	138	2
Genova (15)	Adenoma recurrence	• Vitamin A (6000 IU) + vitamin E (75 mg) + vitamin C (180 mg) + selenium (200 mg) + zinc (30 mg) • Placebo	291	5

Table 1. European chemoprevention studies

The rate of patients with new adenomas is estimated from follow-up study to be 30% after 3 years. As for the polyp growth study, there is a higher rate of patients with an increase in size of the existing adenoma: 40% in patients with an adenoma of less than 5 mm left *in situ* (9). These data give a large number of expected events during follow-up. Thus, a relatively small sample size is sufficient to give the power needed to test the effectiveness of the intervention. The endpoint of intervention studies cannot be invasive cancer itself. This requires an overly large number of subjects and a long study period.

In all European studies, eligible subjects had a complete colonoscopic examination of the large bowel at inclusion in the study (or a left-sided colonoscopy plus a double contrast barium enema in the Genova study), and a complete removal of all polyps, except for the polyp left *in situ* in the Oslo study. Subjects were aged 35–75 years at entry in the ECP (5) and Nottingham studies (7), 25–75 years in the Genova study (8), and 50–75 years in the Oslo study (6). In the Modena study, only the mean age at entry is given: 59.2 years (4).

Non-eligible patients were those with a personal history of colorectal cancer (except in the Oslo study), familial polyposis, an inflammatory large bowel disease, colonic resection or life-threatening diseases.

Chemopreventive agents

In the Modena study, patients were randomized into three groups (4). The first group was given an association of vitamins: vitamin A (30 000 IU), vitamin E (70 mg of α-tocopherol) and vitamin C (1 g); the second group was given 20 g of lactulose; and the third group did not receive any treatment. In the Genova study, included subjects receive either a mixture of antioxidants (selenium, 200 µg; zinc, 30 mg; vitamin A, 6000 IU; vitamin C, 180 mg; vitamin E, 30 mg) or a placebo.

In the three other European studies, one group of patients receive calcium: 2 g/day in the ECP study (corresponding to 13.6 g of calcium glucunolactate and 0.6 g of calcium carbonate: Sandocal, Sandoz), 1.5 g/day in the Nottingham study (as calcium carbonate), and 1.6 g/day in the Oslo study. In the Oslo study, capsules also contain selenium (101 µg), β-carotene (15 mg), vitamin E (75 mg) and vitamin C (150 mg). The daily intake is 10 capsules (6).

In the ECP study a second group of patients receive fibre in the form of ispaghul a husk (Fybogel, Reckitt and Colman). It is administered in a daily dose of 3.8 g as one sachet of orange-flavoured effervescent granules to be diluted in cold water.

Sugar is used as the placebo in the Nottingham study, lactose is used in the Oslo study and sucrose is used in the ECP study. In this last study, two placebos are used, one resembling the calcium supplement and the other resembling the fibre supplement. One-half of the control patients are given the fibre placebo and the other half the calcium placebo.

All these studies have a parallel design. A 2 × 2 factorial design was discussed for the ECP study. It would have had the advantage of estimating the effect of the combination of the two treatments and would have given more power to the study with the same number of participants. This possibility was abandoned because it was not known whether there was a possibility of a negative interaction between calcium and fibre, and because it was thought unlikely that a good compliance could be obtained with a daily intake of five sachets.

Recruitment

Completed or ongoing studies in Europe are relatively small in size. In the Modena study, 255 individuals were randomized into three groups just after polypectomy (4). Among them, 46 had to be excluded because the histological examination revealed no adenoma. Eventually, 70 subjects were included in the vitamin group, 61 in the lactulose group and 78 in the no-treatment group. In the Oslo study, 116 patients were recruited, half in the intervention group and half in the placebo group (6). In some cases a polyp less than 1 cm in diameter

was left *in situ*; in 37 subjects the polyp measured < 5 mm in diameter and in 41 subjects the polyp was 5–9 mm in diameter. In total, 116 patients were included in the study evaluating the recurrence rate of adenomas, and 78 were included in the study evaluating the growth rate. The Nottingham study included 138 individuals (7) and the ECP study included 656 individuals (5): 217 in the calcium group, 219 in the fibre group and 219 in the placebo group. In the Genova study, 291 subjects were randomized of whom 279 were available: 144 in the antioxidant arm and 135 in the placebo arm (8).

Follow-up pattern

The duration varies from one study to the next. In the Modena study, follow-up was performed at the time of the surveillance colonoscopy planned after 6–8 months, 12–18 months and 24–36 months. Contact with the patients was also maintained by telephone calls during and at the end of the follow-up period (4).

In the Oslo study, randomized patients are followed up every 3 months, when they pick up the medication, and a monthly report is sent to the investigator. Non-compliance or poor compliance can therefore be detected and the subjects in question can be contacted for encouragement or better follow-up. A control colonoscopy is performed yearly for 3 years by the same endoscopist (6). Any polyp left *in situ* which reaches 10 mm in diameter is removed. On completion of the study, all polyps will be resected. Intermediate examination of the colon is also planned in the Nottingham study, the final colonoscopy being performed 2 years after the initial one (7).

In the ECP study, all randomized patients are followed up every 6 months (5). At that time, they are interviewed on compliance and observed side-effects, and they are encouraged to continue the study. They are then given their 6-month supply of treatment. The final colonoscopy is performed 3 years after randomization.

Endoscopy is planned for 1 year after randomization in the Genova study and then every other year for 5 years (8).

Secondary end-points

Secondary end-points are summarized in Table 2. In the ECP study, stool samples are collected at entry, after 1 year and after 3 years. In 111 cases, a

Study	Colonoscopy	Stool sample	Cell proliferation	Dietary questionnaire
Modena	0, 1 years	–	–	–
Oslo	0, 1, 2, 3 years	+	–	0, 1, 3 years
ECP	0, 3 years	+	+	0, 3 years
Nottingham	0, 1, 2 years	–	+	–
Genova	0, 1, 3, 5 years	–	–	–

Table 2. Scheme of European chemoprevention studies for colorectal cancer

24-hour collection was obtained. Faecal samples are also collected in the Oslo study 1–2 months after starting the medication, at the first and second year controls and after termination of the medication, making a total of four collections. They will be analysed using the method described by Owen et al. (10) for the detailed quantitative analysis of bile acids and related compounds. These measurements are of importance. Considering the background of the study, it is necessary to document changes in faecal bile acid concentration, giving a unique opportunity to define further the role of faecal bile acids as promoters in colorectal carcinogenesis.

Biopsies from normal mucosa of the upper rectum are taken at the initial and final colonoscopies in the ECP, Oslo and Nottingham studies. They will also be taken during the control colonoscopy after 1 year in the Nottingham study. This part of the study will allow the evaluation of the effect of the intervention on colonic cell proliferation. In the Oslo and Nottingham studies, the biopsies will be processed for Ki-67 analysis, and in the ECP study they will be processed for PCNA analysis.

To interpret the effect of the supplements accurately, it is necessary to take into account a subject's habits vis-à-vis main dietary factors and protective or risk factors that have been related to colorectal cancer. Changes in diet may take place during the course of the study. In the ECP study, identical questionnaires are filled out at the beginning and end of the study. Training of the dieticians in a common interview protocol and a technique for coding the dietary data was one of the important aspects of the research activity in recent years. The dietician who is in charge of this part of the protocol organized training sessions. By correcting training interviews completed by the trainees in their countries, she was able to verify that the understanding of the method and the level of quality of the interviews were high before the real study interviews began. Parallel to this work, a European 'food composition table' was published and a computer program for transforming data from the dietary interviews into simple foods and nutrients was created (11).

In the Norway study, a diet history recall is performed at entry into the study along with a 5-day food registration period with weighing of each food item. In a randomized selection of 29 subjects, dietary recall is repeated after 1 year, as is the 5-day food registration.

Compliance

In the Modena study, 21 subjects (10.0%) did not return for any endoscopic surveillance (2 died and 19 were lost to follow-up), and for 38 subjects (18.2%) the last surveillance colonoscopy was carried out within the 12 months following randomization (4). In 95 subjects (45.5%) the final colonoscopy was performed between 12 and 24 months after entry in the study, and in 55 subjects (26.3%) it was performed after 2 years. Thus only a quarter of the subjects had the third planned colonoscopy. The average trial time was similar in the three groups: 17.5 ± 11.9 months in the vitamin group, 18.2 ± 13.6 months in the lactulose group, and 17.9 ± 13.9 in the untreated group. In addition, 10 patients withdrew from treatment: one in the vitamin group, because of pruritus, three because of lactulose-induced diarrhoea, one because of a stroke, one because of pregnancy and four for various other reasons.

Among the 116 subjects recruited in the Oslo study, 10 drop-outs (8.6%) were registered during the first 18 months: four were due to side-effects of the treatment (abdominal discomfort and unacceptable stool frequency) and a further six were due to inability to comply (6). Compliance with the 1-year colonoscopic control examination was high, at 88.8%.

In the Nottingham study, 138 individuals were randomized and 79 agreed to participate in the study. Four of them withdrew within the first 12 months and 70 completed the study (7).

In the ECP study, 111 subjects have stopped their treatments (16.9%). Most drop-outs occur in the first 6 months (83/111). The main reason is patients not willing to continue taking the treatment over the long study period (39% of the drop-outs). The other main reason is (possible) side-effects (33% of the drop-outs). These patients will be examined at 3 years and the results will be included in the intention-to-treat analysis.

In the Genova study, 55 subjects in the antioxidant group (38.2%) and 51 in the placebo group (37.8%) stopped the treatment (8). At least one endoscopic examination was performed on 150 of the 243 patients who agreed to participate in the study and were followed up for 1 year (62%). The drop-out rate appears to be particularly high in this study. The reasons for non-compliance were unrelated to the treatment, as similar side-effects were observed in both patients assigned to the active compound and those assigned to the placebo.

Results

The only published study is the Modena study (4). Overall, 4 patients in the vitamin group, 9 in the lactulose group and 28 in the untreated group experienced a recurrence of adenomas, i.e. adenomas diagnosed after 1 year of follow-up. In principle, these patients underwent, after the initial endoscopy, a control endoscopy after 6–8 months, with removal of polyps. The percentages of recurrence among those examined after 1 year were 4/49, 9/47 and 28/54 for the vitamin, lactulose and untreated groups, respectively. One of the main limitations of this study was the short follow-up period (only a quarter of the subjects had a colonoscopy after 2 years) and the fact that nearly 30% of randomly assigned patients did not undergo follow-up endoscopy after 1 year. The results nonetheless suggest that antioxidant vitamins, and to a lesser extent lactulose, lower the recurrence rate of adenomas of the large bowel. They have not been confirmed by other studies. Two other studies have found no

effect attribuable to vitamins C and E: a Canadian study testing the effects of vitamins C and E (400 mg daily) on adenoma recurrence (12), and an American study evaluating the effects of vitamin C (4 g daily) and vitamin E (400 mg daily) on adenoma growth in patients with familial polyposis who have undergone colectomy and ileorectal anastomosis (13). Another American study, using β-carotene (25 mg daily) instead of vitamin A, and vitamins C (1 g daily) and E (400 mg daily), found no effect of these vitamins on adenoma recurrence (14) 3 years after a control endoscopy carried out 1 year after randomization. In this context, results of the Genova study will be of interest. Very preliminary results on a small sample of included patients are available: 9 adenomas were detected in the antioxidant group out of 51 subjects who had the 1-year control colonoscopy, and 13 in the placebo group out of 45 subjects who had the 1-year control colonoscopy (15).

In the Oslo study, overall results have been reported concerning the growth and recovery rates of polyps less than 1 cm in diameter that were left *in situ* (16). A reliable *in situ* method for measuring polyp size has been developed in this study (17). Size measurements are performed with a specially designed 1 mm scaled probe. The measurement is made at a rectangular angle from the polyp, which is made possible by the special shape of the probe. A photograph of the polyp with the measuring probe at its side is also taken for easier comparison with the final colonoscopy and later computerized analysis. It has been shown that *in situ* diameter measurements using videoendoscopes and fibre-optic endoscopes were equally reliable and sensitive, and that both instruments can be used interchangeably in follow-up studies of polyp growth (18). Furthermore, the weight of the removed polyp correlated well with the computerized area measurement. In the 103 patients participating in the 1-year control, the recovery rate was higher for polyps of diameter 5–9 mm (94%) than for polyps < 5 mm (81% ; $P < 0.04$), and it was also higher for polyps localized to the colon and the sigmoid colon (91%) than for polyps proximal to the sigmoid colon (78% ; $P < 0.02$). Out of 222 polyps, no change in size was found in 78, and a maximum change of ± 1mm was found in 156. Polyps with an initially recorded diameter of less than 5 mm increased significantly in size, whereas polyps of between 5 and 9 mm were significantly reduced. Overall, 79 new polyps were found in 52 patients. The new polyps were more frequently situated in the right side of the colon than were the initial polyps ($P < 0.01$), and there was a greater occurrence in subjects with multiple polyps than in subjects with only one polyp ($P < 0.04$).

Mucosal proliferation was studied after 1 year in the Nottingham study (7). Supplementation with 1500 mg of calcium produced a significant reduction in the cell proliferation rate, varying from 12.2 at entry to 9.3 after 12 months. There was no significant change in the control group, the corresponding values being 10.6 and 8.9. At 2 years, there was no difference in proliferation between the two groups. Adenoma occurrence rates at 2 years were only 11% in both the calcium and placebo groups. Of the 62 polyps found at 2 years, 43 were metaplastic.

Conclusion

Large bowel cancer is one of the most common cancers and its incidence is increasing in many countries. It thus represents a major public health problem. Primary prevention represents one way of controlling the disease. Large bowel cancer is in most cases the result of a multistage process and at least three steps with separate risk factors can be considered, namely development of an adenoma, growth of the adenoma and, ultimately, cancer. Large bowel carcinogenesis can be modulated at each step of its development. Two European chemopreventive studies have been completed. One of them suggests that a mixture of vitamins A, E and C (and to a lesser extent lactulose) has a protective effect on adenoma recurrence. However, the low compliance rate limits the conclusions of this study. It is also difficult to draw firm conclusions from the Nottingham study which suggests that there is no protective effect of calcium on adenoma recurrence, because the study was too small. Results of ongoing studies evaluating the protective effects of calcium, antioxidants and fibre will be available within 2–3 years.

References

1 Jensen OM et al. Cancer in the European Community and its member states. *Eur J Cancer*, 1990, 26:1167–1256.

2 Berrino F. et all. *Survival of cancer patients in Europe: The EUROCARE study*. International Agency for Research on Cancer, IARC Scientific Publication No. 132. Lyon. (1995)

3 Faivre J, Boutron MC, Quipourt V. Diet and large bowel cancer. In: Zaffia V, Salvatore M, Della Ragione F, eds. *Advances in nutrition and cancer*. Plenum Publishing Corporation, New York, 1994.

4 Roncucci L et al. Antioxydant vitamins or lactulose for the prevention of the recurrence of colorectal adenomas. *Dis Colon Rectum*, 1993, 36:227–234.

5 Faivre J, Boutron MC, Doyon F. The ECP calcium fibre polyp prevention study. Preliminary report. *Eur J Cancer Prev*, 1993, 2:99–106.

6 Hofstad B et al. Growth of colorectal polyps: design of a prospective, randomized, placebo-controlled intervention study in patients with colorectal polyps. *Eur J Cancer Prev*, 1992, 1:415–422.

7 Rooney PS et al. A double-blind, randomized controlled trial of dietary calcium supplementation in individuals with adenomas (one-year results). *Dis Colon Rectum*, 1994, 37:P41

8 Bruzzi P et al. Chemoprevention of metachronous adenoma of the large bowel: a double blind randomized trial of antioxidants. Preliminary results. In: De Palo G, Sporn M, Veronesi U, eds. *Progress and perspectives in chemoprevention of cancer*. Raven Press, New York, 1992:133–140.

9 Hoff G et al. Epidemiology of polyps in the rectum and colon. Recovery and evaluation of unresected polyps two years after detection. *Scand J Gastroenterol*, 1986, 21:853–862.

10 Owen RW, Thompson MH, Hill MJ. Analysis of metabolic profiles of steroids in faeces of healthy subjects undergoing chemodeosycholic acid treatment by liquid gel chromatography and gas liquid chromatography mass electrometry. *J Steroid Biochem*, 1984, 21:593–600.

11 Lieubray-Bornet B et al. *Food composition table for the analysis of European multicentric studies*. Oza, Lyon, 1995.

12 De Cosse JJ, Miller HH, Lesser ML. Effect of wheat fiber and vitamins C and E on rectal polyps in patients with familial adenomatous polyposis. *J Natl Cancer Inst*, 1989, 81:1290–1297.

13 McKeon-Eyssen G et al. A randomized trial of vitamins C and E in the prevention of recurrence of colorectal polyps. *Cancer Res*, 1988, 48:4701–4705.

14. Greenberg ER et al. A clinical trial of antioxidant vitamins to prevent colorectal adenoma. *New Engl J Med*, 1994, 331:141–147.

15 Bonelli L et al. Chemoprevention of metachronous adenomas of the large bowel: a double blind randomized trial of antioxidants. *3rd United European Gastroenterology Week*, Oslo abstract book, 1994:A61.

16 Hofstad B et al. Growth of colorectal polyps: recovery and evaluation of unresected polyps of less than 10 mm, 1 year after detection. *Scand J Gastroenterol*, 1994, 29:640–645.

17 Hofstad B et al. In situ measurement of colorectal polyps to compare video and fiber optic endoscopes. *Endoscopy*, 1994, 26:461–465.

18 Hofstad B et al. Reliability of in situ measurements of colorectal polyps. *Scand J Gastroenterol*, 1992, 27:59–64.

J. Faivre
Registre des Tumeurs digestives (Equipe associée INSERM-DGS), Faculté de Médecine,
7 Boulevard Jeanne d'Arc, 21033 Dijon cedex, France

B. Hofstad
Department of Gastroenterology, Ullevaal Hospital,
0407 Oslo, Norway

L. Bonelli
Unit of Clinical Epidemiology and Trials,
Istituto Nazionale per la Ricerca sul Cancro,
Viale Benedetto XV 10, 16132 Genova, Italy

P. Rooney
Department of Surgery, Queen's Medical Centre,
Nottingham NG7 2UH, United Kingdom

Colon cancer: a USA viewpoint

M. Lipkin

Recent measurements of cell proliferation, differentiation, and gene structure and expression have identified abnormal stages of cell development that are associated with increased susceptibility to cancer. These findings are now being utilized to test mechanisms of action and potential utility of chemopreventive agents both in rodent models and human populations.

In current studies, the rates and distributions of normally and abnormally proliferating and differentiating cells are being measured in rapidly renewing tissues, in order to assay the chemopreventive effects of calcium and other micronutrients. Prostanoids and enzymes involved in their formation are being analysed for chemopreventive effects by measuring arachidonic acid metabolites and inflammatory response. Compounds inhibiting polyamine synthesis are being assayed with ornithine decarboxylase. Chemopreventive inducers of cell differentiation, such as active forms of vitamin D (both naturally occurring and synthetic), are being evaluated for their ability to normalize epithelial cell maturation.

Chemoprevention studies utilizing calcium and several other chemopreventive agents have now progressed from basic measurements to clinical trials. In most of the studies being carried out in which human subjects at increased risk of colon cancer receive oral calcium supplementation, colonic epithelial cell proliferation has now been significantly reduced – these include five randomized clinical trials. These studies have now progressed to short-term human clinical trials, including trials that measure the regrowth of transformed adenoma cells. However, clinical trials measuring the short-term regrowth of adenomas are unable to measure whether chemopreventive agents inhibit early genotoxic events, abnormal cellular metabolic activities involved in tumour promotion over many years, or the progression of adenoma cells to carcinoma.

Thus, more recent studies of chemopreventive agents are being carried out with new standardizations of biomarker assays and additional designs of adenoma clinical trials. These attempt to test the efficacy of chemopreventive agents on human cells, to guide the development of new classes of chemopreventive compounds, and to evaluate their potential for inhibiting human tumours.

Modifications of cell proliferation, differentiation, and gene structure and expression have now identified abnormal stages of cell development that are associated with increased susceptibility to cancer. Measurements of these properties of epithelial cells, referred to as intermediate end-points or biomarkers, are beginning to be carried out, in order to identify the dose response and efficacy of chemopreventive regimens (1, 2).

The abnormal cell development occurring prior to neoplasia is expressed in structural and functional modifications that are relevant to different chemopreventive approaches. The diversity of these cellular abnormalities and the different mechanisms of activity of different classes of chemopreventive agents (3) are resulting in numerous measurements to assay chemopreventive agents and to test them in human populations.

Principles that have guided the development of intermediate end-points for chemoprevention studies include the following.

- Different chemopreventive agents are active during different stages of the evolution of neoplasia.
- This leads to chemopreventive agents having different mechanisms of activity, and to different assays of measurement, i.e. intermediate end-points or biomarkers.
- Many chemopreventive agents have activities via several mechanisms, leading to the development and expression of multiple biomarkers.

Stages in the development of neoplasia, and mechanisms leading to intermediate biomarkers for chemoprevention trials

Fig. 1 summarizes current concepts related to the evolution of stages of neoplasia. Briefly and simply enumerated, normal cells are subjected to events that are genotoxic, resulting in damage to DNA. This damage is normally repaired by extensively functioning DNA repair systems within the cells. With incomplete repair, specific alterations occur in the DNA. Cell proliferation then fixes the modified DNA in initiated cells. Further cell proliferation and events involved in tumour promotion and progression lead to clonal expansion of these cells containing altered DNA, and eventually to the evolution of benign and malignant tumours.

In Fig. 2, the genotoxic events are reviewed in more detail. The damage to DNA can arise both endogenously and exogenously (Fig. 2a). For example, endogenously produced oxidative and alkylation damage can lead to structural changes in DNA with impaired fidelity of DNA repair. Exogenous factors and chronic metabolic and nutritional stresses can similarly contribute to altered DNA (Fig. 2a).

These genotoxic events have been identified by assays (Fig. 2b) including those detecting DNA oxidation and alkylation products excreted into the urine. Other measures of cell toxicity have identified nuclear fragmentation or aberrations. Cell proliferation, as noted above, fixes this altered DNA in initiated cells, and additional mutagenic and related events lead to more advanced abnormalities including micronuclei, sister chromatid exchanges and altered phenotypes.

During stages of tumour promotion and progression (Fig. 2b), further cell proliferation leads to clonal expansion of abnormal cells, accompanied by accumulations of structural gene alterations, and to altered

patterns of gene expression, hyperproliferation, hyperplasia, inflammation aberrant crypt foci and a variety of enzymatic changes, all of which identify intermediate end-points and stages of pre-neoplasia.

Measuring the activity of chemopreventive agents: from basic studies to clinical trials

A summary of current phase II clinical trials in the USA for colon, breast and prostate, in which specific chempreventive agents are being administered, is shown in Table 1. In addition, a dietary intervention trial attempting to lower dietary fat content and increase fibre intake is also underway, measuring colonic adenoma recurrence. A very large clinical trial attempting to inhibit breast cancer incidence by similar dietary modifications, and by increasing calcium intake, is also now getting underway.

In the colon, studies of the activity of calcium on epithelial cell proliferation and differentiation provide an example of how measurements of a chemopreventive agent have progressed from basic to clinical studies (4, 5, 6). Numerous preclinical and clinical studies of calcium's effects have now been carried out, or are underway, including studies:

- *in vitro*, on proliferation and differentiation of epithelial cells and mechanisms of action;
- *in vivo*, on biomarkers of colonic epithelial cell proliferation and differentiation in rodent models and human subjects;
- to inhibit tumour development in rodent models and human subjects.

In vitro, increasing calcium concentration characteristically inhibits cell proliferation and induces differentiation in many types of normal epithelial cells. These include keratinocytes, mammary, oesophageal, bronchial and urothelial epithelial cells. Normal human colonic and other epithelial cells respond to increasing physiological levels of calcium by decreasing proliferation, and this becomes more variable as neoplastic transformation of the cells progresses. In cell and organ cultures, therefore, decreasing external calcium concentration modifies responsiveness to normal external stimuli, and leads to hyperproliferation and impaired differentiation of the cells; normal cell function is usually restored by increasing external calcium concentrations.

In animal models, increased dietary calcium has also modified the proliferation, differentiation and

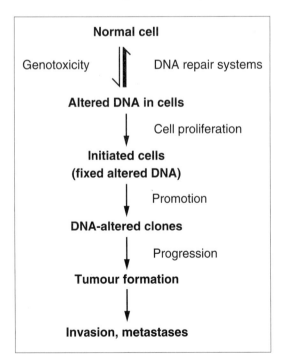

Fig. 1. Stages in the development of neoplasia.

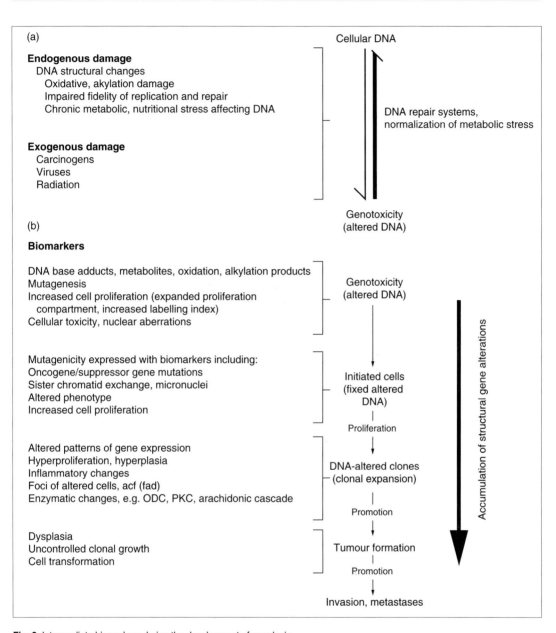

Fig. 2. Intermediate biomarkers during the development of neoplasia.

differential gene expression of colonic epithelial cells. Supplemental dietary calcium decreased colonic cell hyperproliferation when it was induced by bile acids, fatty acids and partial resection of the small intestine in animal models, and calcium also decreased carcinogen-induced colonic tumours in several animal models (Table 2).

In human studies, many previous measurements have indicated that an expansion of the proliferative compartment of the epithelial cells in the colonic crypts has occurred in association with an increased risk of colorectal cancer (7). In most of the human studies carried out, the size of the proliferative compartment has been decreased by increasing the

Table 1. Study design and results of colon cancer intervention trials (USA)[a]						
Authors	Subjects	No.	Treatment	Dose/follow-up	End-points	Results
Completed						
De Cosse	FAP	58	• Fibre + vitamin C + vitamin E • Placebo • Placebo + vitamin C + vitamin E	22.5 g/day 4 g/day 400 mg/day Fibre: 2.2 g/day 4 YEARS	No. of polyps	Reduced with fibre
Reddy	General popoulation, high-fat diet	19	Fibre: • wheat • oats • cellulose • control diet	10 g/day 10 g/day 10 g/day 5 WEEKS	Faecal mutagenic activity	Reduced with wheat and cellulose
Wargovich	Previous adenomas	20	A: –placebo 30 days –Ca 30 days B: –Ca 30 days –placebo 30 days	2 g/day 2 g/day 2 g/day 2 g/day	L.I.[b]	Reduced when switched to Ca
Ongoing						
Alberts	Previous adenomas	1400	Wheat-bran fibre	13.5 g/day 5 YEARS	Adenoma recurrence	
Baron	Previous adenomas	850	Calcium carbonate	1.2 g/day 4 YEARS	Adenoma recurrence	
Giardiello	FAP[c]	15	Sulindac		Cell proliferation, adenomas (no. and volume)	
Graves	Previous adenomas	400	Vegetable- and fruit-rich diet	1 YEAR	Cell proliferation, adenoma recurrence	
Greenberg	Previous adenomas	> 850	β-carotene + vitamin C + vitamin E	30 mg/day 1 g/day 400 mg/day 4 YEARS	Adenoma recurrence	
Meyskens	Previous adenomas	100	Fibre, calcium	3 YEARS	Faecal mutagens	
Mohaban	• Healthy subjects • Colon cancer • Adenomas	20 20 20	β-carotene	30 mg/day (10 mg/day if no effect) 3 MONTHS	 Cell proliferation	

Authors	Subjects	No.	Treatment	Dose/follow-up	End-points	Results
Potter	Previous adenomas	180	Calcium	Two doses 2.5 YEARS	Colonic cell proliferation	
Schatzkin	Previous adenomas (PPT)	2000	Diet: • fats • fruit + vegetables • fibre	< 20% cal 5–8 servings 18 g/kcal 4 YEARS	Mucin change, cell proliferation, adenoma recurrence	
Tilley	Male workers	6000	Screening diet: low-fat, high-fibre	5 YEARS	Cancer incidence	
Wargovich	Previous adenomas	105	Calcium	3 doses (1.5–4 g/day)	Cell proliferation	
Holt	Previous adenomas	60	• Calcium + vitamin D	1.5 g/day (1 YEAR)	Cell proliferation/ differentiation	
		100	• Dietary calcium	1.2 g/day (3 YEARS)	Cell proliferation/ differentiation	
		100	• Calcium + vitamin D	1.5 g/day (3 YEARS)	Polyp growth	

Table 1. (contd.) Study design and results of colon cancer intervention trials (USA)[a]

[a] From Buiatti, Balzi & Barchielli (*11*).
[b] LI, labelling index.
[c] FAP, familial adenomatous polyposis.

calcium intake so that it is above the median level of a Western-style human diet (Table 3). Calcium supplementation has been effective in decreasing epithelial cell hyperproliferation and in correcting abnormal patterns of proliferation in colonic mucosa at increased risk of colorectal cancer. Changes were absent, or less pronounced, when initially low proliferation was present.

Thus, in most of the human studies carried out, both *in vivo* and *in vitro*, increasing the calcium intake to a level slightly above the current human RDA level has decreased colonic epithelial cell proliferation (Table 3). The studies of this effect of calcium now include five randomized clinical trials, four of which resulted in a decrease in hyperproliferation after oral calcium supplementation (8, 9, 10). These four trials included measurements based on the amount of [³H]dThd (8) and BrdU (9) incorporated into proliferating cells, and also measurements of mitotic figures in

colonic crypt epithelial cells (crypt cell production rate; 10).

A recent conference at the NIH (June 1994) on the adequacy of dietary calcium recommended increasing dietary calcium intake in adolescents and several adult groups to 1500 mg/day (which is higher than the current RDA) to reduce the eventual risk of osteoporosis. Although most of the epidemiological, rodent and human studies on calcium intake support this level as a possible means of reducing colon cancer risk, it was recommended that the relationship of calcium intake to colon cancer risk be further studied in clinical trials.

The development of clinical trials to measure adenoma recurrence, and problems to be considered in these trials

As a result of the findings noted above, further clinical trials are currently being planned (or are underway) to evaluate the possible chemopreventive

Table 2. Effects of supplemental dietary calcium on proliferation and differentiation of colonic epithelial cells and on chemical carcinogenesis in rodents		
Cell type	**Calcium effect**	**References[a]**
Colonic	Decreased hyperproliferation induced by deoxycholic acid	Wargovich et al. (1983)
	Decreased hyperproliferation induced by fatty acids	Wargovich et al. (1984)
	Decreased hyperproliferation induced by cholic acid	Bird et al. (1986)
	Decreased hyperproliferation induced by partial enteric resection	Appleton et al. (1986)
	Decreased deoxycholic-acid-induced hyperproliferation (calcium effect blocked by phosphate)	Hu et al. (1989)
	Decreased MNNG-induced hyperproliferation on diet low in fat and calcium	Reshef et al. (1990)
	Decreased hyperproliferation induced by nutritional stress diet (low Ca, vit D; high fat, P)	Newmark et al. (1991)
	Decreased ODC and Tyr K induced by AOM	Arlow et al. (1989)
	Decreased ODC induced by bile acids	Baer et al. (1989)
	Decreased cholic-acid-induced mortality	Cohen et al. (1989)
	Decreased tumour formation induced by partial enteric resection and carcinogen	Appleton et al. (1987)
	Decreased proliferation and tumour formation induced by dietary fat and carcinogen	Pence et al. (1988)
	Decreased intestinal tumours after AOM	Skrypec et al. (1988)
	Decreased colonic tumours induced by AOM	Wargovich et al. (1990)
	Decreased the number of invasive carcinomas after MNU and cholic acid	McSherry et al. (1989)
	Decreased the number of rats with multiple tumours after DMH	Sitrin et al. (1991)
	Unchanged tumour incidence after DMH	Karkara et al. (1989)
	Unchanged tumour incidence after DMH	Kaup et al. (1989)

[a] References given in Scalmati, Lipkin & Newmark (6) and Lipkin (7).

efficacy of a variety of natural substances including calcium. Investigators are attempting to improve the standardization of biomarkers, ranging from cell proliferation to dysplasia, in order to make some of these available for larger studies. In other instances, studies of the effects of chemopreventive regimens on adenoma recurrence are being considered or are underway; these trials will attempt to evaluate whether the regrowth of adenomas will be affected. Clinical trials of this type have great potential for testing the efficacy of chemopreventive agents, but various limitations, some of which are illustrated in Fig. 3, are now known to exist, both in carrying out such trials and in interpreting their results.

A major problem in the design of a clinical adenoma trial is whether it is capable of actually measuring the activity and effect of the chemopreventive agent being tested (Fig. 3). Colonic adenomas develop in the colons of humans over a duration of 20–30 years, evolving and progressing through multiple stages of abnormal cell development from very normal cells to cells that progressively accumulate multiple genetic and metabolic defects which are involved both in genotoxicity and in the initiation, promotion and progression of the cells to tumours. Current clinical trials are now only able to measure the regrowth of small adenomatous tumours which arise from previously transformed adenomatous cells. Furthermore, these measurements can only be carried out during a short 3- or 4-year period, through a small window of observation of short duration that measures the late stage of regrowth of transformed cells (Fig. 3).

Current clinical adenoma trials thus do not measure:

- whether a chemopreventive agent can inhibit genotoxic events from occurring in earlier stages of abnormal cell development;
- whether the agent can inhibit the events involved in tumour promotion to adenomas, which occur over many years;
- whether the agent can inhibit the events involved in the progression of adenomas to carcinomas.

Thus, since adenomas develop over decades, a clinical trial that briefly measures the recurrence of small adenomas over a few years can only measure the possible effect of a chemopreventive agent on mechanisms involved in the rapid regrowth of transformed adenoma cells in late-stage adenoma development. The clinical trial will not measure whether the chemopreventive agent inhibited genotoxic events, cellular metabolic abnormalities involved in tumour promotion or those involved in the progression of adenoma cells to carcinomas.

Naturally occurring potential chemopreventive substances, which are generally safer for use in large populations, often have their major activities in normal or near-normal cells, and have less activity in transformed cells such as adenomas. Different classes of chemopreventive agents also act through different biochemical mechanisms and, in particular, during different stages of tumour initiation, promotion and progression. Therefore chemoprevention studies that use a 3- to 4-year narrow window of observation of adenoma cell regrowth, measuring transformed cells accumulating above the mucosal

Table 3. Effects of supplemental calcium on proliferation and differentiation of colonic cells in human subjects		
Cell type	Calcium effect	References[a]
	Dietary *in vivo*	
Colonic	Decreased hyperproliferation	Lipkin et al. (1985)
	Decreased hyperproliferation	Lipkin et al. (1989)
	Decreased hyperproliferation	Rozen et al. (1989)
	Decreased proliferation	Lynch et al. (1991)
	Decreased proliferation	Berger et al. (1991)
	Decreased proliferation	Wargovich et al. (1992)
	Decreased proliferation	Barsoum et al. (1993)
	Decreased proliferation	O'Sullivan et al. (1993)
	Unchanged proliferation	Gregoire et al. (1989)
	Increased proliferation	Cats et al. (1990)
	In vitro	
Colonic	Decreased proliferation (2mM)	Buset et al. (1986)
	Decreased proliferation (2–4mM)	Appleton et al. (1988)
	Decreased proliferation (2mM)	Arlow et al. (1988)
	Decreased proliferation (2mM)	Buset et al. (1987)
	Decreased proliferation (2mM)	Friedman et al. (1989)
	Protected colonic cells against toxicity of bile acids and fatty acids (5mM)	Buset et al. (1989)
	Increased histone acetylation: cell differentiation (1–2mM)	Boffa et al. (1989)

[a] References given in Scalmati, Lipkin & Newmark (6) and Lipkin (7).

surface, are likely to require potent chemopreventive agents (with potentially higher levels of toxicity), targeted at mechanisms affecting cells in later stages of abnormal development, to achieve a rapid inhibitory effect on the regrowth of transformed adenoma cells. In order to design clinical trials that can accurately test the utility of diverse classes of chemopreventive agents, chemoprevention studies should therefore incorporate the following information into the design of the clinical trial.

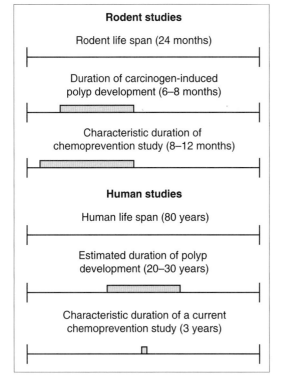

Fig. 3. Rodent and human life spans, showing the typical periods during which carcinogen-induced colonic tumours develop and during which chemoprevention studies are carried out. Previous chemoprevention studies in rodents have characteristically administered the agent to be tested over a large part of the rodent's life span, beginning at an early age. In humans, adenomas develop over a long duration, evolving through multiple stages of abnormal cell development from normal cells to cells that progressively accumulate multiple genetic and metabolic defects which are involved in genotoxicity and in the initiation, promotion and progression of the cells to tumours. However, current clinical adenoma trials are only able to measure the regrowth of small adenomatous tumours during a late stage of abnormal cell development as the transformed cells accumulate above the surface of the colonic mucosa.

1 The specific stage of abnormal cell development that is being measured.

2 Whether or not the known activity of the agent previously observed to be effective in preclinical studies is being measured in cells during the stage of adenoma development being studied.

3 Whether this activity corresponds to mechanisms that are being measured in the proposed adenoma clinical trial.

Other errors in adenoma studies include the fact that adenomas are often missed during examinations, and poor compliance after several years. Thus, in a single colonoscopy, 10% or more of small adenomas may not be detected. These considerations, as well as others that occur in large-scale clinical trials which are not addressed here, will need to be considered when planning and carrying out human adenoma trials with chemopreventive agents.

References

1 Lipkin M, Levin B, Kim Y, eds. Intermediate biomarkers of precancer and their application in chemoprevention. *J Cellular Biochem*, 1992, 16G:1–196.

2 Boone CW, Kelloff GJ, eds. Quantitative pathology in chemoprevention trials: standardization and quality control of surrogate endpoint biomarker assays for colon, breast, and prostate. *J Cellular Biochem*, 1994, Sl9:1–293.

3 Cancer chemoprevention. In: Wattenberg L, Lipkin M, Boone CW, Kelloff GJ, eds. CRC Press, 1992:1–630.

4 Calcium, vitamin D and prevention of colon cancer. In: Lipkin M, Newmark H, Kelloff GJ, eds. CRC Press, 1992:1–435.

5 Newmark HL, Lipkin M. Calcium, vitamin D, and colon cancer. *Cancer Res*, 1992, 52: 2067s–2070s.

6 Scalmati A, Lipkin M, Newmark H. Calcium, vitamin D, and colon cancer. 1992, *Clin Appl Nutr*, 2:67–74.

7 Lipkin M. Biomarkers of increased susceptibility to gastrointestinal cancer: New application to studies of cancer prevention in human subjects. *Cancer Res*, 1988, 48:235.

8 Wargovich MJ et al. Calcium supplementation decreases rectal epithelial cell proliferation in subjects with sporadic adenoma. *Gastroenterology*, 1992, 103:92–97.

9 O'Sullivan KR et al. Effect of oral calcium supplementation on colonic crypt cell proliferation in patients with adenomatous polyps of the large bowel. *Eur J Gastroenterol Hepatol*, 1993, 5:85–89.

10 Barsoum GH et al. Reduction of mucosal crypt cell proliferation in patients with adenomatous polyps by dietary calcium supplementation. *Br J Surg*, 1992, 79:581–583.

11 Buiatti E, Balzi D, Barchielli A. *Intervention trials of cancer prevention*. IARC Technical Report No. 18. Lyon, International Agency for Research on Cancer, 1994.

M. Lipkin
Memorial Sloan-Kettering Cancer Center,
New York, NY 10021, USA

Why did antioxidants not protect against lung cancer in the Alpha-Tocopherol, Beta-Carotene Cancer Prevention Study?

J.K. Huttunen

The Alpha-Tocopherol, Beta-Carotene (ATBC) Lung Cancer Prevention Study was a randomized, double-blind, 2×2 factorial design, primary prevention study testing the hypothesis that α-tocopherol (50 mg/day) and β-carotene (20 mg/day) supplements reduce the incidence of lung cancer and possibly other cancers. A total of 29 133 male smokers aged from 50 to 69 years participated in the study (mean duration 6.1 years) accumulating 169 751 follow-up years. The study failed to demonstrate a protective effect of antioxidant supplements on lung cancer, and raised the possibility that β-carotene might be harmful in this population. Possible explanations for the unexpected result are that an incorrect dose was used, the duration of the study was too short or the study population was inappropriate; the possibility of bias is less likely, as the study was logistically a success.

Introduction

Epidemiological studies have provided strong and consistent evidence that high intakes of fruits and vegetables are associated with a lowered risk of cancer (1). The relationship is strongest for cancers of the oral cavity, oesophagus, lung and colon. Fruits and vegetables contain several nutrients which may protect against cancer (1, 2). They are the principal sources of three antioxidant vitamins, vitamin C, β-carotene and vitamin E. Other compounds in fruits and vegetables that may have anticarcinogenic activity include flavonoids, isothiocyanates, indoles, folate and fibre.

Final proof that any compound has a role to play in the prevention of human cancer can only be obtained from a sufficiently large controlled trial. Several ongoing intervention trials are testing the hypothesis that β-carotene or vitamin E are protective against cancer in humans (3). This paper discusses the central findings of the Alpha-Tocopherol, Beta-Carotene Cancer Prevention Study (ATBC; 4, 5), a large, double-blind, placebo-controlled primary prevention trial, jointly sponsored by the Finnish National Public Health Institute and the United States National Cancer Institute.

Design and results of the ATBC study

The ATBC study involved 29 133 male smokers between 50 and 69 years of age living in south-western Finland. The participants were randomly assigned to one of the four daily supplement regimens: synthetic DL-α-tocopherol (50 mg), synthetic β-carotene (20 mg), both α-tocopherol and β-carotene, or placebo. Data on the main confounders confirmed that the assignment was a random one. The mean duration of the study was 6.1 years (range 5–8 years). A total of 21% of all participants stopped smoking during the study. Furthermore, 9061 participants (31.1%) left the study for various reasons, including death. Altogether, 3570 deaths occurred during the trial.

Cases of lung cancer were identified through the Finnish Cancer Registry. To enhance the ascertainment of cases of lung cancer, a chest X-ray was obtained during a study visit every 28 months and on each participant's exit from the study. Information on morbidity unrelated to cancer was obtained from the Finnish National Hospital Discharge Registry. Deaths and causes of death were identified from the National Death Registry.

Contrary to the initial hypothesis, an excess cumulative incidence of lung cancer was observed in the β-carotene group after 2 years, and this increased progressively thereafter, resulting in an 18% difference in incidence (474 versus 402) by the end of the study ($P < 0.01$). Lung cancer was 2% lower in the vitamin E-supplemented group (433 versus 443, $P = 0.8$). There was no interaction between the two supplements in their effect on lung cancer. The participants who received α-tocopherol had fewer cancers of the prostate than those who did not (99 versus 151).

Total mortality was 2% higher ($P = 0.6$) in the α-tocopherol groups than in the groups that received no α-tocopherol, and 8% higher ($P = 0.02$) among the participants who received β-carotene than among those who did not. There were more deaths due to lung cancer, ischaemic heart disease and ischaemic and haemorrhagic stroke among recipients of β-carotene.

Consistent with several other reports (6), the incidence of lung cancer in the placebo group was significantly higher among the subjects in the lowest quartile of baseline serum vitamin E and β-carotene than among those in the highest quartile. An inverse correlation was observed between the risk of lung cancer and the dietary intake of both β-carotene and vitamin E at baseline.

Comments

The results of the ATBC study provide no evidence that supplements of β-carotene or α-tocopherol afford protection against lung cancer. On the contrary, the data have raised the possibility that β-carotene might increase the risk of lung cancer and ischaemic heart disease death in smokers.

Several explanations for the unexpected outcome of the ATBC study should be considered. Bias as a cause of the results seems unlikely. No differences were observed in risk factors of cancer or cardiovascular disease between the treatment groups at baseline, and the changes in these characteristics during the study were similar, with the obvious exceptions of serum α-tocopherol and β-carotene levels. Compliance was excellent and the drop-out rate was lower than expected. The total number of lung cancers observed during the study was in good agreement with the power calculations. The essentially complete case ascertainment (incidence of and mortality from cancer, total mortality and disease-specific mortality) assured the comparability of trial treatment results.

According to the scientific rationale, antioxidants are likely to be of value during the early stages of carcinogenesis (7). The Finnish study may have failed to detect beneficial effects of antioxidant vitamins because supplementation began at a relatively late point during the chain of events that leads to clinical lung cancer. Long-term follow-up of the trial cohort using mortality and disease registers is of paramount importance, as it will provide information on the effects of antioxidants on early phases of the disease processes.

An important consideration in the interpretation of the data is the dose of antioxidants used. For α-tocopherol, the dose selected for the study

(50 mg/day) represents an approximately fivefold excess over the mean dietary intake of the source population, and clearly exceeds the dietary intakes that have been associated with low cancer risks in epidemiological studies. The dose for β-carotene (20 mg/day) is 6–10 times that of the mean dietary intake in European and North American populations, and approximately three times greater than the highest quintile of intake associated with the lowest risk of lung cancer in epidemiological studies. However, because of differences in bioavailibility and metabolism, the observed changes in serum levels of α-tocopherol and β-carotene were different: a 1.4-fold increase was observed in serum vitamin E in subjects supplemented with α-tocopherol, while the change in β-carotene level in subjects supplemented with β-carotene was 16-fold.

It has been suggested that the α-tocopherol dose used in the study may have been too small to have any substantial impact on lung cancer or ischaemic heart disease (8). It should be noted, however, that the dose clearly exceeded the dietary intakes that have been associated with cancer protection in epidemiological studies. Therefore, a benefit should have been detected, if the associations observed in epidemiological studies are causal. Conversely, the dose of β-carotene may have been high, as the synthetic formulation used in the study has a particularly high bioavailability. Thus, the possibility that a beneficial effect would have been detected with a dose closer to physiological intakes cannot be totally excluded.

Several authors (8, 9, 10) have speculated that the unexpected results might be due to the peculiarities of the trial population, e.g. smoking, diet, alcohol consumption or genetic characteristics. This interpretation seems unlikely; the fat and alcohol intakes were in the same range as those in most Western populations, and there are no indications that Finns differ substantially from other northern European or North American populations with regard to cancer susceptibility or metabolism of fat-soluble vitamins. On the other hand, these characteristics might very well explain the conflict between the results of the Finnish study and those of the Linxian Study (11) conducted in a Chinese population with a very different diet and lifestyle.

The ATBC study observation of a higher incidence of lung cancer and a higher mortality from ischaemic heart disease in subjects receiving β-carotene are contrary to the results of two other intervention trials (*11, 12*). As we have discussed earlier, there are no known mechanisms of toxic effects, no data from studies in animals suggesting β-carotene toxicity, and no evidence of serious toxic effects in humans (*13*). Therefore, the increased incidence of lung cancer and increased mortality from ischaemic heart disease in subjects supplemented with β-carotene may well be due to chance.

In summary, the Finnish–American ATBC Cancer Prevention Study failed to demonstrate a protective effect of supplemental α-tocopherol and β-carotene in male smokers aged 50–70 years. Possible explanations for the unexpected result are that an incorrect dose was used, characteristics of the study population were inappropriate, or the duration of the study was too short; bias is less likely to have been a cause, as the study population was large, intervention groups were well balanced, treatment compliance was excellent and case ascertainment was complete. Further conclusions on the beneficial or harmful effects of antioxidant vitamins on lung cancer must await the results of other ongoing clinical trials (*14, 15, 16*) and further follow-up data from the ATBC study becoming available.

References

1 Block G, Patterson B, Suber A. Fruits, vegetables and cancer prevention: a review of the epidemiological evidence. *Nutr Cancer*, 1992, 18:1–29.
2 Doll R, Peto R. The causes of cancer. New York, Oxford University Press, 1981.
3 Greenwald P. Experience from clinical trials in cancer prevention. *Ann Med*, 1994, 26:73–80.
4 The Alpha-Tocopherol, Beta-Carotene Cancer Prevention Study Group. The effect of vitamin E and beta carotene on the incidence of lung cancer and other cancers in male smokers. *N Engl J Med*, 1994, 330:1029–1035.
5 The Alpha-Tocopherol, Beta-Carotene Cancer Prevention Study Group. The Alpha-Tocopherol, Beta-Carotene Cancer Prevention Study: design, methods, participant characteristics, and compliance. *Ann Epidemiol*, 1994, 4:1–10.
6 Rautalahti M, Huttunen JK. Antioxidants and carcinogens. *Ann Med*, 1994, 26:435–442.
7 van Poppel G. Carotenoids and cancer: an update with emphasis on human intervention studies. *Eur J Cancer*, 1993, 9:1335–1344.
8 Blumberg J, Block G. The Alpha-Tocopherol, Beta-Carotene Cancer Prevention Study in Finland. *Nutr Rev*, 1994, 52:242–250.
9 Hennekens CH, Buring JE, Peto R. Antioxidant vitamins – benefits not yet proved. *N Engl J Med*, 1994, 330:1080–1081.
10 Buring JE, Hebert P, Hennekens CH. The Alpha-Tocopherol, Beta-Carotene Lung Cancer Prevention Trial of Vitamin E and beta-carotene: the beginning of the answers. *Ann Epidemiol*, 1994, 4:75.
11 Blot WJ et al. Nutrition intervention trials in Linxian, China: supplementation with specific vitamin/mineral combinations, cancer incidence, and disease-specific mortality in the general population. *J Natl Cancer Inst*, 1993, 85:1483–1492.
12 Gaziano JM et al. Beta-carotene therapy for chronic stable angina. *Circulation*, 1990, 82:Suppl.III,III–201.
13 Bendich A. The safety of beta-carotene. *Nutr Cancer*, 1988, 11:207–214.
14 Steering Committee of the Physicians' Health Study Research Group. Final report on the aspirin component of the ongoing Physicians' Health Study. *N Engl J Med*, 1989, 321:129–135.
15 Thornquist MD et al. Statistical design and monitoring of the Carotene and Retinol Efficacy Trial (CARET). *Control Clin Trials*, 1993, 14:308–324.
16 Buring JE, Hennekens CH. The Women's Health Study: summary of the study design. *J Myocard Ischemia*, 1992, 4:27–29.

J.K. Huttunen
National Public Health Institute,
Mannerheimintie 166,
FIN-00300 Helsinki,
Finland

Chemoprevention of lung cancer: the β-Carotene and Retinol Efficacy Trial (CARET) in high-risk smokers and asbestos-exposed workers

G.S. Omenn*, G. Goodman, M. Thornquist, S. Barnhart, J. Balmes,
M. Cherniack, M. Cullen, A. Glass, J. Keogh, D. Liu, F. Meyskens, Jr,
M. Perloff, B. Valanis and J. Williams, Jr

Lung cancer is the most common cancer and the leading cause of cancer-related deaths in the world, with an estimated 900 000 new cases and 785 000 deaths per year (1, 2). In addition to primary prevention of cigarette smoking, certain occupational exposures and household radon exposures, chemoprevention strategies are urgently needed, given the tens of millions of people already exposed and the poor results of treatment for lung cancer.

CARET (β-Carotene and Retinol Efficacy Trial) is a multicentre, two-armed, double-masked randomized chemoprevention trial being conducted in six study centres in the United States, the aim of which is to test whether oral administration of β-carotene (30 mg/day) and retinyl palmitate (25 000 IU/day) can decrease the incidence of lung cancer in high-risk populations, i.e. heavy smokers and asbestos-exposed workers. The intervention combines the antioxidant action of β-carotene and the tumour-suppressor mechanism of vitamin A. CARET randomized 1 845 participants in its 1985–1988 pilot phase plus 16 469 participants between 1989 and 1994; of the 18 314 total participants, 4 060 are asbestos-exposed males, and 14 254 are smokers and former smokers (44% female). Accrual has been completed and the safety profile of the regimen to date has been excellent. We estimate that CARET will have accumulated 108 800 person-years by October 1997 and will be capable of detecting a 23% reduction in lung cancer incidence in the two populations combined. CARET will then be able to detect 27%, 49%, 32%, 35% and 35% reductions in the smoker, female smoker, male smoker, asbestos-exposed and former smoker subgroups, respectively. CARET will also have

*Correspondence: G.S. Omenn, School of
Public Health and Community Medicine,
University of Washington, SC-30, Seattle, WA 98195,
USA.

substantial power to detect possible chemopreventive effects on coronary heart disease plus sudden cardiac death, cataract extraction rates and prostate cancer incidence. CARET is highly complementary to the ATBC (Alpha-Tocopherol, Beta-Carotene) study in Finland, the Physicians' Health Study (β-carotene alone) and the Women's Health Study (β-carotene, vitamin E and aspirin) in the NCI (National Cancer Institute) portfolio of major cancer primary chemoprevention trials. Media coverage in April 1994 of the surprising, unexplained and adverse findings in the ATBC trial led 577 CARET participants to stop taking the CARET capsules, 3.8% of all active participants.

Potentially attractive agents for next-generation lung cancer chemoprevention trials may include N-acetyl-l-cysteine and oltipraz, 9-cis retinoic acid and other retinoids, and difluoromethylornithine (DFMO).

Introduction

Lung cancer is the leading cause of cancer-related death among both men and women in the United States, accounting for approximately 28% of cancer deaths and 6% of all deaths. An estimated 153 000 Americans died of lung cancers in 1994 (3). Despite aggressive therapy, the 5-year survival remains disappointing, at approximately 15%. In recent years, lung cancer incidence has begun to decline among men in the developed countries. However, smoking-related lung cancer incidence has continued to rise among women. Meanwhile, lung cancer incidence is rising dramatically in developing countries (4). Lung cancer surpassed breast cancer in the mid-1980s as the leading cause of cancer-related death among women in the United States, so it is important to study chemoprevention of lung cancer in women as well as in men.

Primary and secondary prevention of lung cancer is eminently feasible. The primary risk factor, cigarette smoking, is well established (5, 6). Prevention of smoking and smoking cessation occupy deservedly prominent places throughout the world in national plans to reduce age-adjusted cancer death rates. Unfortunately, the prevalence of smoking in the United States did not decline in 1992 (7). In combination with those efforts, cancer control strategies aimed at preventing the development or progression of tumours in people who already have histories of cigarette smoking are essential. In the United States, 29% of men and 25% of women in the 45–64 age group are current smokers (7), and at least 40% of men and 20% of women aged 45–64 years are former smokers (8). The latency period offers a major opportunity to intervene to delay or prevent cancers in these high-risk populations.

Interacting synergistically with cigarette smoking in relation to lung cancer risk is exposure to respirable fibres of asbestos (9, 10). In the case of asbestos-related cancers, primary prevention efforts should be redoubled to improve occupational exposure standards and protective equipment, and to develop substitute materials for asbestos. Secondary prevention is important since an estimated four million workers had significant exposure to asbestos in shipyards and related activities during World War II (11), leading to 4000–6000 excess lung cancer deaths per year at present (11, 12).

β-carotene, vitamin A, and synthetic and naturally occurring retinoids have attracted wide interest as possible chemopreventive agents against lung cancer, based on observational epidemiology and animal studies (13, 14, 15). Eleven out of 15 prospective, and 10 out of 17 retrospective, epidemiological studies have found a statistically significant association between low dietary or serum β-carotene and increased risk of lung cancer (15). In human intervention studies, retinoids have reduced the incidence of micronuclei in buccal smear cells (16) and sputum cells (17): 13-cis retinoic acid reduced the incidence of second primaries in patients treated successfully for head and neck cancer (18); retinyl palmitate (300 000 IU/day) increased the time to relapse or new primary tumour among patients with stage I lung cancer (19); and retinol (25 000 IU/day) reduced the incidence of squamous cell, but not basal cell, skin cancer in patients with actinic keratosis (20). However, retinol, β-carotene and 13-cis retinoic acid had no effect on patients with previous skin cancers (20, 21, 22). Furthermore, randomized trials with etretinate (23), β-carotene plus vitamin A (24), and 13-cis retinoic acid (25) had no effect on sputum atypia (23, 24) or on biopsy metaplasia (25). Such mixed results in studies of intermediate end-points and prevention of recurrences demonstrate the necessity of large, randomized chemoprevention trials in various high-risk populations.

The exact mechanisms of chemopreventive activity are unclear, but β-carotene is an electron-scavenging antioxidant diminishing late stage cell surface lipid peroxidation, and retinol enhances the differentiated state of epithelial cells, including bronchial epithelium, presumably through binding to specific nuclear receptor proteins (the RAR and RXR series) which regulate gene expression, cell differentiation, proliferation and apoptosis (26). Both β-carotene and retinoids enhance some aspects of the human immune system (27).

In the early 1980s, the United States National Cancer Institute (NCI), impressed with the evidence pointing to the potential chemopreventive effects of β-carotene, launched three major prevention trials: β-carotene (50 mg BASF on alternate days) alone was administered in the Physicians' Health Study (in a 2×2 design with aspirin; PHS) involving 22 071 United States male physicians at low risk of lung cancer (28); β-carotene (20 mg Roche) plus vitamin E (50 mg) was administered in the Alpha-Tocopherol/Beta-Carotene (ATBC) trial involving 29 113 male smokers in Finland (29); and β-carotene (30 mg Roche) plus vitamin A (25 000 IU) was administered in the β-Carotene and Retinol Efficacy Trial (CARET) based in Seattle, involving 18 314 male and female current or former smokers and male asbestos-exposed workers (30, 31). ATBC was completed and reported in 1994, as will be discussed below and also by Dr Huttunen in his paper, which is included in this monograph; PHS results are expected in 1996 and CARET results are expected in 1998.

The primary aim of this paper is to provide a substantial progress report for CARET. In addition, we will comment on the implications of the ATBC results reported from Finland in 1994 and on future directions for phase III chemoprevention trials against lung cancer.

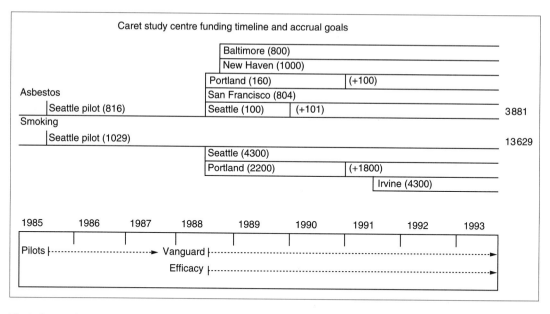

Fig. 1. Schema for recruitment of participants in CARET.

Development and organization of CARET

CARET is a randomized, double-masked, placebo-controlled chemoprevention trial involving two groups of adults at high risk of lung cancer: men and women aged 50–69 years with a history of at least 20 pack-years of cigarette smoking; and men aged 45–69 years with evidence of extensive occupational exposure to asbestos and a history of cigarette smoking. CARET is evaluating the efficacy and safety of a daily combination of 30 mg of β-carotene plus 25 000 IU of retinyl palmitate (*30, 31*). CARET has been built up in stages, as shown in Fig. 1, beginning in 1985 with two successful pilot studies, as part of the Cancer Prevention Research Program of the Fred Hutchinson Cancer Research Center and the University of Washington School of Public Health and Community Medicine in Seattle. CARET's efficacy phase received funding in July 1988 for additional recruitment at the Seattle study centre and for new study centres in Baltimore, New Haven, San Francisco and Portland. Final expansion began in southern California in mid-1991 at the Irvine study centre. Accrual of 18 314 participants was completed in September 1994. Participants will take study vitamins up to October 1997.

A steering committee sets CARET policy, reviews progress, approves protocol modifications and has final approval of publications and any ancillary studies. An external 'Safety and Endpoints Monitoring Committee' (SEMC) meets with the PI and Coordinating Center statisticians twice each year to review the semi-annual progress report, to discuss the progress of the study in detail, and to recommend continuation of the study.

Study structure and stepwise recruitment

The two CARET pilot studies randomized 1029 current and former smokers and 816 asbestos-exposed workers between June 1985 and August 1988. Male and female smokers recruited via mailings to 29 928 subscribers to King County Medical Blue Shield were randomized in a 2 × 2 factorial phase II trial of 30 mg β-carotene and/or 25 000 IU retinol daily versus placebo (*32*). Men occupationally exposed to asbestos were recruited from federal and state workers' compensation programmes, selected occupational medicine and pulmonary physicians, plaintiffs' attorneys, the Navy Asbestos Medical Surveillance Program, and major unions in the Puget Sound area into a two-arm trial of the combination of 15 mg β-carotene and 25 000 IU retinol daily versus placebo (*33*). Among asbestos pilot participants, 16% were never smokers and 36% had stopped smoking more than 15 years before enrolment; in order to recruit a higher-risk population, we restricted eligibility criteria for subsequent CARET recruitment to eliminate these two groups, requiring smoking within the 15 years before randomization as a criterion.

Participants in both pilots demonstrated good adherence to the daily vitamin regimen, as measured by capsule consumption rates. The only significant difference in monitored symptoms and signs between intervention arms was yellow coloration of the skin, generally mild, with β-carotene. Median β-carotene concentration in the two smoker arms receiving β-carotene increased 12-fold by 4 months and reached a plateau at that level; for the asbestos active arm (half the dose), the concentrations increased eightfold. In the retinol-containing arms, median retinyl palmitate values increased fourfold and serum retinol concentrations increased slightly (32, 33).

At the end of the two pilot studies, all active pilot participants were asked to continue in the long-term efficacy trial, as the 'vanguard' cohort. All those who were in active arms in the pilot studies had their dosage changed to 30 mg β-carotene and 25 000 IU retinyl palmitate daily (identical to the CARET efficacy intervention); those on placebo continued on placebo. As of 31 December 1994, 1552 (84%) of the pilot participants had made the transition; 1153 (74%) of these vanguard participants were still active, while 155 (10%) had died. All 1845 pilot participants are followed for efficacy end-points.

As shown in Table 1, CARET randomized 4060 asbestos-exposed workers and 14 254 heavy smokers, obtaining a grand total of 18 314 participants, which exceeded accrual goals (Fig. 1). To give an idea of the scale of recruitment required, randomization of the 16 469 efficacy participants required 1 441 479 recruitment letters, 45 588 completed screening phone calls and 22 116 enrolment visits. The yield was low since it was not possible to screen most recruitment lists for smoking-eligible individuals.

Randomization was based on a permuted blocks algorithm with random block size and equal allocation to the two arms, stratified by study centre and

Population/ study centre	85–86	86–87	87–88	88–89	89–90	90–91	91–92	92–93	93–94	94–95	Total
Asbestos-exposed workers											
Baltimore	–	–	–	–	187	454	165	3	4	–	808
New Haven	–	–	–	–	267	385	238	131	3	–	1024
Portland	–	–	–	–	23	98	100	73	14	–	308
San Francisco	–	–	–	–	206	291	253	96	8	–	845
Seattle pilot	190	444	182	–	–	–	–	–	–	–	816
Seattle efficacy	–	–	–	–	14	23	119	85	4	–	245
Total	**190**	**444**	**182**	**–**	**697**	**1251**	**875**	**388**	**33**	**–**	**4060**
Heavy smokers											
Irvine	–	–	–	–	–	–	328	1590	2110	196	4224
Portland	–	–	–	67	778	1295	998	912	207	–	4257
Seattle pilot	378	499	152	–	–	–	–	–	–	–	1029
Seattle efficacy	–	–	–	50	1205	690	1456	1155	149	–	4482
Asbestos spouses[b]	–	–	–	–	–	–	22	16	1	39	–
Grand total	**568**	**943**	**334**	**117**	**2680**	**3236**	**3657**	**4067**	**2515**	**197**	**18 314**

Table 1. CARET recruitment (final; number randomized by year of randomization[a])

[a]Years run from July to June to match funding schedule. Pilot recruitment 1985–88; efficacy recruitment May 1989 – September 1994.
[b]Additional recruitment of household members who are smoker-eligible at asbestos study centres (Baltimore 9, New Haven 18, San Francisco 12).

exposure population. The unit of randomization was the household, to guard against household members taking the wrong vitamin type, while (hopefully) enhancing adherence in pairs. Approximately 10% of randomized participants are members of the same household as other CARET participants. The intra-household correlation in lung cancer incidence is estimated to be 0.03, based on the observed distribution of lung cancer risk factors in our household pairs and a relative risk of 1.5 for the effect of passive smoking (34). At randomization, a sample of 12.5% of efficacy participants was identified for quality assurance on serum analyses (additional 10 ml blood). An independent 10% sample of participants across all strata were selected to be cohort members of the case–cohort design (35) used for analyses of serum α- and β-carotene, retinol, retinyl palmitate and α-tocopherol. Serum is obtained annually from vanguard participants and biennially from efficacy participants; beginning in 1994, all active participants were sampled for whole blood (in tubes and on filter paper) for later DNA probe assays of biomarkers.

Participant characteristics

The Coordinating Center carefully monitors participant baseline characteristics to ensure the eligibility of participants, to check the balance of risk factors between intervention arms, and to reassess periodically the sample size requirements based on the participants' risk factors against the CARET design parameters (30). In the combined pilot and efficacy cohorts, the asbestos-exposed and smoker participants at randomization had mean ages of 57 and 58 years; 38% and 66% were current smokers; and the mean pack-years were 41 and 49, respectively. Mean years since smoking cessation were 19 and 7 for the pilot and efficacy asbestos-exposed populations, respectively, and 3 for both smoker populations. Of the asbestos-exposed participants, 44% were positive by chest X-ray for asbestos-related changes and had a protocol-defined high-risk-trade work history, while 22% had a positive X-ray only, and 34% had a high-risk-trade history only. Among those with positive X-rays, 27% showed changes in the parenchyma only, 41% in the pleura only, and 32% had both pleural and parenchymal changes. Mean years from first asbestos exposure to randomization was 35 years.

CARET has been successful in recruiting women: 44% of the total heavy smoker population is female. This is especially noteworthy since women (aged 50–69 years) are more likely never to have been smokers and since female smokers smoke less than their male counterparts (7, 8). For example, in the three-county recruitment area for the Seattle study centre, 46% of the female population aged 50–69 years are 'never smokers' compared with 26% of males (based on unpublished pooled control data from Fred Hutchinson case–control studies). Minorities make up about 12% of the asbestos-exposed population and 4% of the smoker population (asbestos: 8% African-American, 2% Hispanic, 1% Asian/Pacific Islander, 1% other; smokers: 2% African-American, 1% Hispanic, 1% Asian/Pacific Islander, 1% other). Systematic data on minority representation were not available from any of the recruitment sources used. Relatively high yields from local minority populations were achieved by Baltimore and San Francisco. Portland, Seattle and Irvine, which are located in areas with low percentages of age-eligible minorities, did mount extensive efforts to recruit minorities.

Follow-up (and monitoring)

The literature on the design and conduct of primary prevention trials (36) focuses mainly on recruitment and on close-out and analysis, with little attention to the middle phase of extended follow-up, which may comprise more than half the total duration of the trial (37). Monitoring participants for end-points and safety, assisting participants in smoking cessation, maintaining participants' interest in and enthusiasm for the trial, and monitoring the trial's progress are the major foci of the follow-up phase of CARET.

Follow-up and symptom monitoring

In the first year after randomization, efficacy participants are contacted four times, by telephone at 3 and 9 months and by visits to the study centre at 6 and 12 months. In subsequent years, efficacy participants are contacted by telephone at 4 and 8 months after the randomization anniversary date and they make an annual visit to the study centre. Since effects are likely to depend on the duration of exposure, any side-effects of the study vitamins should appear in the vanguard cohort first. The active vanguard group is monitored more closely, with semi-annual visits, additional questions on symptoms, and annual analysis of

Table 2. Status of participants: pilot and vanguard cohorts as of 31 December 1994			
	Asbestos-exposed participants	Heavy smoker participants	Total
Pilot study			
Randomized	816	1029	1845
Became inactive or died during pilot	140	251	391
Vanguard cohort			
Made transition	708 (87%)	844 (82%)	1552 (84%)
– while active in pilot	676	777	1453
– by reactivation	32	66	98
Became inactive or died since transition	203	243	446
– currently inactive or dead	18	214	399
– reactivated and alive	18 29	47	
Pilot participants			
Currently active	523 (64%)	630 (61%)	1153 (62%)
Currently inactive and alive	179 (22%)	266 (26%)	445 (24%)
Dead	114 (14%)	133 (13%)	247 (13%)
Vanguard participants			
Currently active	523 (74%)	630 (75%)	1153 (74%)
Currently inactive and alive	118 (17%)	126 (15%)	244 (16%)
Dead	67 (9%)	88 (10%)	155 (10%)

non-fasting serum for SGOT, alkaline phosphatase, cholesterol and triglycerides. In vanguard participants, the development of a symptom exceeding the predefined threshold grade or an increase in hepatic enzyme markers triggers the CARET symptom management protocol (32). All threshold grade symptoms are reviewed by the study centre PI, as are all episodes of non-adherence attributed to side-effects. Every 6 months, the external SEMC reviews, by coded intervention arm, the mean grade and proportion of participants who exceed threshold grades for each monitored symptom and liver function test, as well as the number of participants becoming inactive due to symptoms.

No consistent clinically significant excess of any of the 13 monitored symptoms and signs has been observed to date, except mild skin yellowing. As of 31 December 1994, 968 full-dose symptom management cases have been completed (170 vanguard and 798 efficacy): 921 resulted in a return to full-dose, 28 in a return to half-dose, and 19 in a removal from the study vitamins.

Since we contact CARET participants often and ask detailed questions about symptoms, we conducted a survey in June 1992 of negative and positive impacts of this questioning on participants. About 97% of 400 participants reported that they liked the phone calls or were neutral; 83% thought we should maintain the present frequency; 56% reported that they liked the symptom assessment questions in the interviews; 71% thought the content of the symptom questions was just right; and 87% recognized the health-monitoring aspect of the phone calls, which we have reinforced in our multifaceted retention activities.

Smoking cessation

At each visit after randomization, study centre interviewers actively encourage current smokers to quit smoking and former smokers to maintain smoking cessation, via referrals and self-help materials. At the last analysis, up to 31 December 1994, 29% of efficacy participants who were current smokers at the first visit had accepted smoking cessation packets, 14% of efficacy smokers at baseline

Table 3. Status of participants: efficacy cohort as of 31 December 1994

	Active		Inactive		Number of participants randomized
	Continuously active	Reactivations	Alive and inactive	Dead	
Asbestos-exposed participants					
Baltimore	678 (83%)	1 (<1%)	86 (11%)	48 (6%)	813
New Haven	881 (86%)	3 (<1%)	96 (9%)	44 (4%)	1024
Portland	259 (84%)	2 (<1%)	39 (13%)	8 (3%)	308
San Francisco	676 (79%)	17 (2%)	125 (15%)	36 (4%)	854
Seattle	208 (85%)	1 (<1%)	31 (13%)	5 (2%)	245
Total	**2702 (83%)**	**24 (<1%)**	**377 (12%)**	**141 (4%)**	**3244**
Heavy smoker participants					
Irvine	3495 (83%)	4 (<1%)	694 (16%)	31 (<1%)	4224
Portland	3344 (79%)	32 (<1%)	734 (17%)	147 (3%)	4257
Seattle	3822 (81%)	51 (1%)	671 (14%)	161 (3%)	4705
Household members[a]	38 (97%)	0 (0%)	1 (3%)	0 (0%)	39
Total	**10 699 (81%)**	**87 (<1%)**	**2100 (16%)**	**339 (3%)**	**13225**
All efficacy participants	13 512 (82%)		2477 (15%)	480 (3%)	16469
Pilot/vanguard/efficacy	14 665 (80%)		2922 (16%)	727 (4%)	18314

[a]Members of asbestos-exposed participants' households randomized at Baltimore, New Haven and San Francisco.

reported abstinence at 24 months, while 4% of former smokers had resumed smoking. Our analyses indicate that the effects of smoking cessation on sample size projections are negligible (30). In both efficacy and vanguard cohorts, an additional 5–6 % of baseline current smokers have achieved abstinence each year after year 2.

Retention: active rates and vitamin adherence

Retention begins with an informed participant and supportive staff. The CARET quarterly newsletter provides project-specific and general health and social support studies. Side-effect fact sheets and letters to personal physicians have been helpful. Mugs, magnets, pins and certificates of appreciation have been presented to participants and appear to be appreciated. Tables 2 and 3 show the percentage of randomized participants who were active (alive and receiving study vitamins), alive and inactive, or deceased as of 31 December 1994. Using statistical methods for functions of multiple Kaplan–Meier curves developed by Pepe (38), we estimate for living efficacy participants that, at 4 years post-random-

ization, 87% of those who were asbestos-exposed and 79% of heavy smokers are active. The most common reasons for becoming inactive are health issues other than monitored symptoms or cancer (cited by 33% of inactive efficacy asbestos-exposed participants and 28% of inactive efficacy heavy smoker participants) and development or fear of monitored symptoms (14% and 13%, respectively). The pilot/vanguard participants continue to show high long-term active rates: at 5 years after transition to vanguard, 86% of living asbestos-exposed participants and 86% of heavy smokers are active.

In light of the long duration of CARET, the Coordinating Center has developed a standardized procedure for approaching inactive participants to encourage them to restart the study vitamins (except for those few participants for whom capsules were stopped according to the symptom management protocol); this procedure begins 6 months after inactivation. As of 31 December 1994, 150 efficacy participants and 156 pilot/vanguard participants have become active again.

CARET end-points: efficacy

Lung cancer is the primary CARET disease end-point. Secondary end-points are mesothelioma, all other cancers (except non-melanoma skin cancers) and death. All pilot/vanguard and efficacy participants, including inactive participants, are followed for end-points. Primary sources for initial notice of end-points are study participants or their next of kin; secondary sources are state and SEER (surveillance, epidemiology and end results) cancer registries in California, Connecticut, Maryland, Pennsylvania, Washington and Virginia, the Kaiser Permanente patient database in Portland, state Boards of Health and the National Death Index. CARET's 'Endpoints Committee' has developed stringent criteria for the ascertainment and review of end-point cases. Up to 31 December 1994, 838 cancer end-point cases and 560 death end-point cases had been closed by the Endpoints Committee, and another 248 cancer and

167 death end-point cases are pending completion of data collection and review (Tables 4 and 5). The lung cancer yield is in close agreement with our projections, at an incidence rate of 4.9 lung cancers/1000 person-years (Table 4). The 286 participants diagnosed with lung cancer exceed one-half of the total of 519 participants projected for February 1998 (Table 6).

CARET was designed to have 80% power to detect a 23% reduction in lung cancer risk in participants receiving active study vitamins compared with those receiving placebo (30, 39); such a difference corresponds to a 33% 'maximal potential chemopreventive effect' before dilution by such factors as competing causes of death, time-lag to full effect, imperfect adherence to the regimen, and intake of equivalent vitamins in the diet or supplements of placebo-arm participants. With 4060 asbestos-exposed participants and 14254 heavy smokers,

Table 4. Cancer end-points[a]: pilot/vanguard and efficacy cohorts as of 31 December 1994

Primary site[b]	Pilot/vanguard		Efficacy		
	Asbestos-exposed participants	Heavy smokers	Asbestos-exposed participants	Heavy smokers	Total
Lung cancer	27	44	52	163	286
Mesothelioma	11	0	4	1	16
Unknown primary, lung involvement	0	0	1	3	4
Other cancer (prostate)	83 (40)	102 (30)	130 (57)	442 (103)	757 (230)
Number of participants	119	140	179	596	1034
Number of end-points	125	151	191	619	1086
Closed	116	130	151	441	838
Open	9	21	40	178	248
Person-years of follow-up for lung cancer	5920	7653	10875	32847	57296
Lung cancer incidence rate ($\times 10^3$/person per year)	4.6	5.7	4.8	5.0	5.0
95% confidence interval[c]	(3.2, 6.7)	(4.2, 7.7)	(3.7, 6.3)	(4.3, 5.8)	(4.5, 5.6)

[a]Closed and open end-points combined. For end-points which are not yet closed, primary site is based on *Form 31–Initial Notice of Endpoint*. Only CARET end-points are included (e.g. basal and squamous cell skin cancers and recurrences are excluded).
[b]Participants are represented no more than once in the counts of each primary site; however, a participant may be counted for more than one primary site. Note: four participants had two lung cancer primaries each, 19 participants had a lung primary and another type of primary, and 20 participants had multiple non-lung primaries.
[c]Confidence intervals are based on the normal approximation to the Poisson distribution.

Table 5. Death end-points[a]: pilot/vanguard and efficacy cohorts as of 31 December 1994

| Cancer diagnosis[b] | Pilot/vanguard | | Efficacy | | |
	Asbestos-exposed participants	Heavy smokers	Asbestos-exposed participants	Heavy smokers	Total
Lung cancer	20	38	32	87	177
Mesothelioma	10	0	2	1	13
Unknown primary, lung involvement	0	0	1	3	4
Other cancer (prostate)	26 (5)	31 (5)	22 (1)	60 (4)	139 (15)
No cancer	58	64	84	188	394
Total deaths	**124**	**133**	**141**	**339**	**727**
Closed	106	120	106	228	560
Open	8	13	35	111	167
Person-years of follow-up for death	5944	7705	10923	329757	57548
Mortality rate ($\times 10^3$/person per year)	19.2	17.3	12.9	10.3	12.6
95% confidence interval[c]	(16.0, 23.1)	(14.6, 20.5)	(10.9, 15.2)	(9.3, 11.5)	(11.7, 13.6)

[a]Closed and open cases combined. For cases which are not yet closed, cancer diagnosis is based on *Form 31–Initial Notice of Endpoint.*
[b]Participants who had both a lung cancer and another cancer are counted under lung cancer.
[c]Confidence intervals are based on the normal approximation to the Poisson distribution.

CARET will achieve this target power by October 1997 (year 10), according to current projections. CARET will be capable of detecting 27%, 49%, 32%, 35% and 35% reductions in the subgroups of smokers, female smokers, male smokers, asbestos-exposed participants and former smokers, respectively. For secondary end-points, CARET has 80% power to detect a population risk reduction of 64% for mesothelioma, 27% for prostate cancer, 13% for all-cause mortality, and 19% for mortality from coronary heart disease and sudden cardiac deaths. We will conduct exit contacts, conclude follow-up and close the study centres by mid-1998. The additional follow-up gained during that close-out period is estimated to increase the power of CARET to 84% to detect a 23% reduction in risk, provided any risk reduction continues after withdrawal of the study vitamins. Naturally, an extension of the follow-up period would increase the power further, so long as participation and follow-up of end-points are sustained and any risk difference is maintained.

We monitor the use of vitamin supplements. Only 2% of CARET participants are taking supplementary β-carotene and 1% take over 5500 IU of vitamin A; average doses are far below the study dosage. We do not adjust the trial duration calculations to take account of differences between the arms in dietary intake of β-carotene and retinol, but we will examine the effect of dietary intake in the analyses planned.

From the beginning, we have explored the possibilities for conducting ancillary intermediate end-point trials within CARET, which would offer the advantage of being able to correlate the end-point with the 'true' end-point, lung cancer. However, there are currently no validated intermediate end-points for lung cancer. Sputum atypia was investigated by McLarty (24) in the Tyler, Texas, cohort of asbestos-exposed men, using the CARET regimen as an intervention, without a direct tie to clinical end-points.

During the long course of CARET, evidence from observational studies has emerged associating β-carotene and often retinol (as well as vitamins E and C) with significantly lower risks of cardiovascular mortality (40, 41) and cataracts (42). Therefore, we

Table 6. Projected person-years of follow-up and numbers of lung cancers

Population and cohort	Active group			Placebo group		
	Person-years of follow-up	No. of lung cancers	No. of weighted lung cancers[a]	Person-years of follow-up	No. of lung cancers	No. of weighted lung cancers
Pilot asbestos	4200	16	15	4100	20	19
Pilot smokers[b]	8000	32	29	2700	13	12
Efficacy asbestos	10400	69	58	10300	90	77
Efficacy smokers	37400	122	100	37400	157	133
Total[c]	60000	239	202	54500	280	241

[a]Weighted by $w(t) = \min(t/y, 1)$, where t is the time since randomization and y is the time-lag to full effectiveness (2 years).
[b]Active arm has larger number of person-years, reflecting 3:1 ratio in the pilot heavy smoker group.
[c]The sum of numbers in the column may differ from total due to rounding.

have added protocols for examination of these end-points in CARET. We expect to have 80% power to detect a 19% reduction in the combined end-point of fatal myocardial infarction plus sudden cardiac death. A special history-taking introduced in 1993–1994 has yielded, up to 31 December 1994, diagnoses of cataracts in 1254 participants and cataract extractions in 412 participants after randomization. We expect cataract extractions to be an end-point collected by history only. We are currently contacting participants' ophthalmologists to confirm the date and ascertain the type of cataract. In baseline analyses, we also have reports of 909 people diagnosed with cataracts and 398 participants with extractions pre-randomization. We expect to have 80% power to detect a 19% reduction in cataract extraction rates.

CARET end-points: safety

The vanguard and efficacy cohorts are monitored routinely for 13 symptoms (skin redness, dryness, itching and yellowing; lip chapping, bone pain, nosebleeds, vomiting, frequency of bowel movements, weight loss, headaches, anxiety, depression), which can all be side-effects of β-carotene or vitamin A. These are graded according to the CARET symptom assessment scale (32). In addition, non-fasting blood samples are obtained annually from vanguard participants for analysis of SGOT, alkaline phosphatase, triglycerides and total cholesterol. Given the large number of participants, the study has a high power to detect a difference between intervention arms in reported side-effects and serum analyte concentrations. For example, we will have 99% power to detect whether 4 years of supplementation with the CARET study vitamins increases the mean skin redness grade by (as little as) 0.04 on a scale from 0 to 5; the threshold grade which triggers symptom management is 4. All participants are asked at baseline and at each follow-up visit if they have been told by a doctor that they have had any of 33 specific health-related conditions (or any other). During the past year, we have reported reassuring information that the CARET regimen of 30 mg β-carotene plus 25 000 IU retinyl palmitate does not depress serum α-tocopherol levels (43) or trigger hypertriglyceridaemia, even in persons with elevated levels at baseline (44).

Establishing the safety of any chemopreventive agent is essential, especially since participants (and future users) are healthy volunteers without cancers, and not patients (45). Even for the high-risk participants in CARET, the chance of having lung cancer diagnosed is less than 1/100 per year. Thus, it is important to avoid significant side-effects, both objective and subjective.

Trial monitoring

Risk factor monitoring and accrual pace can, of course, inform adjustments in study design, including sample size and trial duration. In the case of CARET, the study centres exceeded the recruitment targets by over 800 participants, and the adherence of participants to taking their study vitamins continues to exceed design assumptions, enhancing study power. Smoking cessation, which has been encouraged, has been shown to have negligible impact on power (30, 37). Intensive monitoring of data quality, and maintenance of staff and participant enthusiasm are important features. To this end, we are conducting several subprojects; these include randomized tests examining the participants' subjective responses as well as any impact on adherence due to retention items, such as certificates or pins as tokens of appreciation at milestone dates, and individualized feedback from computerized analyses of the CARET food frequency questionnaire. We also give CARET mugs and CARET magnets, involve participants in a quarterly newsletter, and organize participant advisory committees. During the long middle-phase, opportunities may arise for investigation of additional hypotheses within the same dataset or with additional data that can be readily collected, as illustrated above for cardiovascular disease and cataracts. Finally, if additional trials are anticipated, it is wise to prepare the ground and seek the funding for such trials before key staff start looking for new challenges, and before close-out and analysis demands full attention.

Analytical plans

The primary analysis, based on intention to treat, is designed to test for differences between intervention arms in the incidence of lung cancer, using a stratified, weighted log-rank statistic. The weight function incorporates a linear down-weighting of events occurring in the first 2 years post-randomization to compensate both for a time-lag to full intervention effect and for undetected cancers that may be present at enrolment.

Secondary analyses of CARET data will include the following.

●The effect of the CARET regimen on lung cancer incidence in defined subgroups (defined by exposure population, age and sex).
●The effect of the CARET regimen on the incidence of mesothelioma, prostate cancer and other cancers; on mortality rates from all causes and from coronary heart disease, both overall and within subgroups; and on the incidence of cataract extractions.
●The extent to which any effect of CARET agents on primary or secondary end-points is associated with achieved serum levels, non-dietary intake of retinol and β-carotene (both from the study vitamins and from supplementary vitamins), and dietary intake of retinol and β-carotene.
●The effect of the CARET regimen on symptoms and signs that are potential side-effects of vitamin A or β-carotene.
●The relationship between CARET efficacy end-points and baseline factors, such as smoking history, diet, age, sex, occupational history and spirometric and X-ray findings.
●The sensitivity of the primary analysis to the choice of weighting for the time to full effect.

To characterize our asbestos-exposed population further, we will model lung function (as measured by biennial spirometry) against intervention assignment, time since randomization, cumulative dose, smoking history, dietary factors, age, other medical conditions, X-ray findings, and symptom reports using generalized linear models. In both populations (asbestos-exposed and smoker), we will analyse the effect of long-term supplementation on the serum concentrations of the vitamins, evaluate the changes that have occurred with the transition to vanguard (change in vitamin dose and combination, and the resultant change in serum concentration of vitamins), and evaluate the relationship between the participants' characteristics (such as age, sex, smoking, asbestos exposure, alcohol intake and diet) and serum retinoid and carotenoid concentrations.

Analyses planned prior to the conclusion of CARET will include the following areas: recruitment and baseline characteristics of CARET participants; recruitment strategies – comparison of yields by mailing sources and mailing types, based primarily on the systematically varied experience of the Portland study centre; early predictors and reasons for participants becoming inactive, according to risk factors, behavioural responses, serum levels and publication of the ATBC trial results; quality assurance in CARET; measures to enhance adherence and retention; longitudinal analyses of the effects of study vitamins on serum triglycerides and vitamin E levels; bias in self-reported food intake; and use of the household as the unit of randomization. Additional analyses planned for the completion of follow-up include the following areas: enhancing adherence in long-term prevention studies; correlation of lung cancer risk with putative biological markers in stored samples; generalization of findings to populations at risk of lung cancer; relationship between fibrosis at baseline and subsequent lung cancer and total cancer risk in asbestos-exposed individuals; comparison of asbestos-exposed groups across different high-risk trades and/or recruitment sources; and effect of intervention on spirometry findings in asbestos-exposed individuals.

Each study centre is encouraged to undertake certain ancillary studies, with the approval of the steering committee. For example, the Yale group is evaluating retinol, total carotenoid and α-tocopherol levels in lung tissues obtained from CARET participants who develop cancer and undergo lung resection, and in bronchoalveolar lavage macrophages (Redlich et al., unpublished). The aims are to determine the range of micronutrient stores in the lung, the potential of lavage macrophage measurements to serve as risk factor biomarkers for lung cancer, the responsiveness of lung and lavage macrophages to the administration of CARET study vitamins, and the effects of CARET study vitamins on non-study micronutrient levels. They are investigating a strong association between the presence of bronchial metaplasia and inflammatory lavage cells in asbestos-exposed subjects (46) for possible mediation by transforming growth factor β, interleukins 6, 8 and 11, platelet-derived growth factor and scatter factor, which may be regulated by retinoic acid (47).

We also have CARET-wide committees for clinical investigation and for development of biomarker studies. Current candidates for biomarker studies include the polymorphic biotransformation enzyme systems thought to be active and important in pulmonary carcinogenesis – cytochrome P450 enzymes 1A1 and 2D6, glutathione-S-transferase-mu, epoxide hydrolase and N-acetyl-transferase – plus p53 and other potential mediators of proliferation.

Assessing the implications of the ATBC results

The most important challenge to the conduct of CARET during 1994 was the reporting of results from the ATBC trial in Finland (29). As is now well known, neither vitamin E (at 50 mg/day) nor β-carotene (at 20 mg Roche β-carotene/day) had any beneficial effect on lung cancer, total mortality or cardiovascular mortality. Such a result could easily have been attributed to inadequate dose, inadequate duration of follow-up or inadequate power to detect a modest effect. However, the analysis of β-carotene results showed an adverse effect on lung cancer risk (OR = 1.18, with 95th CI = 1.03–1.36) and total mortality (OR = 1.08, CI = 1.01–1.16), with excess cardiovascular deaths (653 versus 586).

Had the ATBC results been favourable, as was expected, one can only wonder at the awkwardness, or even the impropriety, of maintaining the participants in the Physicians' Health Study and CARET on placebo arms, or beginning the Women's Health Study of β-carotene and vitamin E (48) with a placebo arm. Ironically, the ATBC results, which were shared with every participant in CARET via individual letters received on the day before publication in the *New England Journal of Medicine*, have forced us to work hard to retain participants who are worried about being in the active arm! We have been scrupulously candid in describing the ATBC results, noting that they are unexpected in light of observational and experimental animal work, but making clear that the study was well designed and well conducted, and represents the most important test to date of the hypothesis that increasing β-carotene intake could reduce lung cancer risk. We also pointed out that completion of CARET is essential to address the new questions that the ATBC results present. Written communications with participants in the immediate aftermath of the ATBC publication were reviewed in advance by the CARET SEMC and by individual institutions' 'Human Subjects Review Committees'. Oral communications were scripted accordingly. Special efforts have been made to explain the ATBC findings to CARET staff and co-investigators and to welcome and discuss all of their questions.

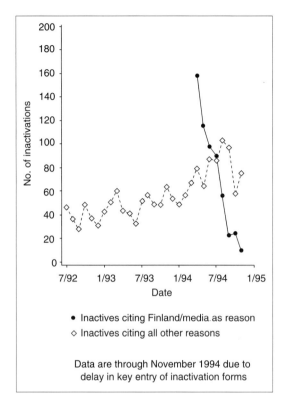

Data are through November 1994 due to delay in key entry of inactivation forms

Fig. 2. Number of inactivations in CARET per month: July 1992 – November 1994

As discussed above, we monitor reasons why participants become inactive. After the publication of ATBC results on 14 April 1994, we recorded that 577 participants (3.8% of active participants) became inactive, citing ATBC results as the reason. As shown in Fig. 2, the effect was prompt, even more prompt than indicated in this figure, which records the date when CARET staff learned of the inactive status; in most cases, the participant stopped taking the study capsules earlier. We are no doubt vulnerable to further inactivations should there be another wave of media publicity about the ATBC as additional papers are published, or should there be other adverse information.

Media attention in the United States was intense, reflecting high interest in cancer prevention and aggressive promotion of β-carotene and other vitamin supplements for prevention of cancers and other health problems. In fact, the United States Congress was under intense pressure to deny the

Food and Drug Administration the authority to require evidence to support the health claims of vitamin manufacturers! More than 200 Members of Congress (out of a total of 435) were co-sponsors of a bill sought by the vitamin manufacturers and their customers. Headlines in April were a curious mix of surprise ('Vitamins Don't Make Smokers Cancer-Proof', 'Benefit of Vitamins Disputed') and alarm ('β-Carotene Causes Cancer'). We are interested to know more about the media coverage and reactions of trial participants in Europe. Apparently, sales of β-carotene were unaffected in Europe, except for the Scandinavian countries where they fell sharply (Dr Dietrich Hornig, Roche/Basel, personal communication).

No plausible explanation for the ATBC findings has been put forward yet, although chance ($P = 0.01$ for lung cancer; $P = 0.02$ for total mortality) might still account for the adverse effects associated with β-carotene, as compared with a null result (but not as compared with a highly favourable effect). If β-carotene were somehow directly or indirectly toxic at high doses, one would expect that the excess mortality and excess lung cancer cases would be in those with the highest tertile of serum β-carotene values when they were assayed after 3 years of treatment; such was not found (Albanes et al., personal communication). However, an association of high alcohol intake with lung cancer was identified (Albanes et al., personal communication). We have analysed our CARET data for potential alcohol effect and have found none so far, using either CARET quartiles of self-reported alcohol intake or ATBC cutpoints, which are much higher. Perhaps β-carotene caused a relative deficiency of some other antioxidant or protective endogenous substance; serum vitamin E levels were measured and were unaffected in the β-carotene arm (as in CARET; *43*). It is conceivable that the β-carotene contained some unrecognized carcinogenic contaminant, but none has been proposed. We did learn, to our surprise, that the Roche β-carotene used in our 1985–1988 pilot period contained about 10% α-carotene (now confirmed by Roche, V. Singh, personal communication).

Perhaps Finns are different from Americans... But the baseline analysis of ATBC findings showed the expected inverse relationship between serum and dietary β-carotene and subsequent lung cancer and total mortality, so we can dismiss one of the main criticisms in a recent critique (*49*). There is much post hoc speculation that the very deliberate choice of high-risk smokers – most at risk and with the greatest potential benefit – might not have been a wise choice, since 6 years of intervention might be too little too late to modify lifelong accumulated risks. However, relative risks (if not absolute risks) of lung cancer and absolute risks of coronary heart disease certainly decline after smoking cessation (*50*). Advocates of vitamin E benefit point out, with some justification, that the dosage used (50 mg) and the serum levels of α-tocopherol achieved (about 35% increase over baseline) were quite modest, which is true. However, the evidence that higher doses might be needed arose somewhat unexpectedly, years after ATBC was initiated, in a study of dietary intake, which was essentially negative for vitamin E benefit except in those taking vitamin E supplements (*51*). Furthermore, the ATBC result of increased haemorrhagic stroke with vitamin E must be weighed against using much higher doses.

About all that can be concluded at this time is that we must await the results of the Physicians' Health Study, CARET and the Women's Health Study (all primary prevention studies), and the Women's Antioxidant Cardiovascular Study (*41*) and other secondary prevention trials, at which time there will be an adequate base of information to guide health promotion efforts and regulatory review of the efficacy and safety of vitamin supplements (*52*). We must even be cautious about our conclusions concerning the direct benefits of high intakes of vegetables and fruits. We must challenge observational epidemiologists to put forth specific *a priori* hypotheses about the parameters, foods and biomarkers that are expected to be associated with disease outcomes. It is painfully true that we don't know which of the many vegetables and fruits studied, which nutritional constituents or which features of the people studied account for the striking, but diverse, associations observed (*41, 44, 53*). The most recent study of vegetable and fruit intake in relation to cardiovascular disease risk (*40*) included an interesting analysis of food categories, which pointed again to β-carotene as the leading specific candidate. The suspicion that there is an adverse effect associated with β-carotene can only be dispelled with additional results from the ongoing randomized trials.

Future directions for cancer chemoprevention

The reactions to the ATBC results reinforce the importance of various challenges inherent in chemoprevention trials. When is there enough information to justify a randomized trial, yet not enough compelling evidence that the 'window' has passed and the proposed intervention is accepted as general guidance?

Should or can diets be studied using random assignment? Does the evidence from observational epidemiological studies of diets guide us adequately in selecting agents to be administered in a supplement? What dose is likely to be maximally efficacious, and yet safe? What dose is sufficient? Is the dose chosen in order to address a deficiency state or to act pharmacologically regardless of baseline status? If it is the former, should prospective participants be screened to exclude those who are not deficient, and what criteria should be used to define 'deficient'? What are the most appropriate features for trial participants? Are high-risk individuals (elderly, smokers, occupationally exposed) likely to be more responsive or less responsive? Is the benefit–risk ratio likely to be much lower in low-risk participants? Are effects likely to be different in pre-menopausal versus post-menopausal women? Will the administration of one agent in substantial doses cause disequilibrium with other endogenous or dietary protective factors? Does smoking or alcohol substantially alter the pharmacodynamics of micronutrients? How long would it take to begin to see a difference in incidence of cancers or cardiovascular end-points? What duration of intervention is needed in order to shift risk profiles and incidence significantly? How confident can we be of power estimates? Is it ethical to recruit participants to a trial when a benefit is commonly assumed, for example if the public is already advised through official dietary guidelines to increase their intake of vegetables and fruits? Will it be feasible to sustain the trial if persuasive evidence of benefit – or adverse effect – arises from other sources?

First, we must be certain to gain maximal information from the major trials already conducted. It is wise that the National Cancer Institute (NCI) and the Finnish National Public Health Institute have extended the follow-up (without further treatment) of ATBC and that the Physicians' Health Study has been extended periodically. These studies,

CARET and other trials must examine specific hypotheses about potential favourable and unfavourable effects, to the extent that existing and obtainable data permit. Their serum and DNA banks must serve as sources for testing biomarkers and potential intermediate end-points; if such end-points can be identified and validated, a whole new generation of studies would be expedited.

Second, we need cooperative analyses of data from the present studies and the same in the future. Real-time comparisons of data items on questionnaires, laboratory assay methods and results, pharmaceutical agents or diets, and participant characteristics can facilitate interpretation of similarities and differences in results that would otherwise remain topics for speculation.

Third, we should encourage IARC and NCI and other responsible bodies to continue to examine basic cancer biology, epidemiological findings and laboratory findings on natural products for new leads to chemopreventive agents. Dozens of agents are already under investigation in the NCI phase I and phase II programmes (54, 55). As possible candidates, some of these agents may soon be in the limited window of opportunity for randomized, large-scale, phase III chemoprevention trials, i.e. where there is sufficient justification to recruit participants and to invest the considerable sums required for a reliable study, but the agent is not yet widely used despite a strong scientific basis.

Table 7. Cancer chemopreventive agent candidates for which NCI has clinical development plans[a]

N-acetyl-l-cystine	Ibuprofen
Aspirin	Oltipraz
Calcium	Piroxicam
β-carotene	Sulindac
DHEA analogue 8354	Tamoxifen
2-difluoromethylornithine	Vitamin D3 and
(DFMO)	analogues
Finasteride Proscar	Vitamin E
18b-Glycyrrhetinic acid	
N-4-hydroxyphenyl retinamide	
(4-HPR)	

[a]Kelloff et al. (59).

Strategies have been defined for seven common tumour sites: colorectal, prostate, lung, breast, bladder, oral cavity and cervix, generally relying upon pre-malignant, *in situ* or intraepithelial lesions as end-points. The United States National Cancer Institute has clinical development plans for, at the least, the agents listed in Table 7 (56).

Fourth, it is timely to examine certain specific classes of agent as potential next-generation phase III agents against lung cancer. Retinoids are of particular interest, given the extensive favourable animal data and the portfolio of human intervention trials with retinol, retinyl palmitate, and N-(4-hydroxy-phenyl)retinamide. We should probably see the results from the present studies before launching additional phase III studies with related agents. However, there is a vast array of retinoid compounds, and work with the endogenous ligand 9-cis retinoic acid and its analogues may suggest new approaches. RAR-selective compounds are potent inhibitors of cell proliferation and induce differentiation, which RXR-selective compounds do not; on the other hand, activation of RXRs is essential for induction of apoptosis (57).

Oltipraz (4-methyl-5-pyrazinyl-3H-1,2-dithiol-3-thione) is an interesting prospect. This agent is approved and widely used to treat patients with schistosomiasis. Oltipraz has been chosen recently as the chemopreventive agent in a trial against primary hepatocellular carcinoma in Qidong, China. It is known to induce glutathione-S-transferase activity, which may be protective against certain carcinogens involved in lung cancer, as well as other cancers. GST activity might be a useful biomarker, and GST-mu genotype and phenotype may be a useful risk factor. This synthetic dithiolthione is structurally related to compounds found in cruciferous vegetables. It has been shown to act at both post-initiation and initiation stages of carcinogenesis (55). It has been effective against colon, bladder, lung and breast cancers in animals. There may be marked individual variation in the human metabolism of this agent, which should be characterized (possibly related to P450/CYP 2D6 polymorphism). Phase II trials of oltipraz are directed at Chinese patients with previous respiratory tract cancers and those at high risk of liver cancer because of aflatoxin B1 exposures and chronic hepatitis B infection; additional phase II trials in breast, bladder and lung cohorts are planned for commencement in 1995.

Oltipraz has shown synergistic chemopreventive activity with DFMO (difluoromethylornithine) in mouse bladder, with β-carotene in hamster lung, with 4-HPR in mouse bladder and hamster lung, and with carbenoxolone in rat mammary systems. It has inhibited the development of foci of aberrant crypts in rat colon and of AFB1-induced enzyme-altered foci in rat liver. However, there may be serious problems with side-effects, ranging from phototoxicity (finger pain, reddish discoloration of fingernails, increased sunburn and paraesthesias) to gastrointestinal upsets.

Another promising, already approved pharmaceutical, used as a mucolytic agent, is N-acetyl-l-cysteine, which serves as a precursor for intracellular synthesis of cysteine and glutathione, and thereby increases glutathione levels, by a mechanism entirely different from Oltipraz. Based on striking inhibitory effects *in vitro* and *in vivo*, this compound is under study for prevention of second primary lung cancers in the European project Euroscan (58) in combination with retinyl palmitate. N-acetyl-l-cysteine also has anti-inflammatory properties, inhibits prostaglandin synthesis, inhibits ODC activity and may enhance DNA repair (59). For 1995, NCI is considering a phase II trial of NAC at 1.4 g/m^2 per day (compared with 600 mg/day in Euroscan) to investigate modulation of squamous metaplasia/dysplasia, ploidy, p53, PCNA and EGFR biomarkers in chronic smokers with or without prior smoking-related cancers. It is thought that NAC may be effective at lower doses against bladder and colon cancers.

Another promising agent proposed for advanced human trials is DFMO, 2-(difluoromethyl)ornithine. DFMO is a potent irreversible inhibitor of ornithine decarboxylase (ODC), which catalyses a crucial step in the synthesis of polyamines, from ornithine to putrescine. Thus, ODC inhibition should inhibit cell proliferation. The lung is not considered a high-priority site for DFMO trials, although DFMO significantly inhibited lung tumour formation in hamsters when offered in combination with 4-HPR, β-carotene or both (60).

Other agents require extensive human safety studies before consideration for phase III trials, as well as more phase I/II characterization of efficacy, mostly with surrogate intermediate end-points and biomarkers. It is important to remember that most chemical agents have multiple actions, not just a particular effect first studied in cell culture or animal models (7). A broad array of mechanisms is under investigation, and many good candidates can be expected to emerge from this work. An NCI/FDA Working Group has spelled out extensive guidance for development and clinical testing of chemopreventive agents (59).

Conclusion

Large-scale cancer prevention trials represent major challenges in concept, design, execution and analysis. CARET is a smoothly functioning, well managed study with enthusiastic participants and established quality control procedures which have now been adopted by several other large chemopreventive trials. We are on track to achieve the power designed for CARET by late 1997. If β-carotene and retinyl palmitate can give a 23% observed reduction in lung cancer incidence in CARET, this result would extrapolate to a saving of 34 000 lives per year in the United States and 180 000 lives per year worldwide.

Prevention remains a powerful strategy for control of the common cancers. Behavioural, nutritional and pharmacological prevention trials are still in the early stages of development. Designs of prevention trials must account for characteristics of the nations within which they are conducted. For example, follow-up of participants is greatly facilitated by the existence of national population registries; although CARET uses the SEER registries where possible, coverage of cancer diagnoses is not complete, so CARET must also rely on self-reporting of cancer by participants. The Physicians' Health Study uses self-reporting by participants entirely, relying on the fact that the participants are physicians. The ATBC trial was able to draw on complete cancer data from the Finnish national health registry, resulting in reduced costs for follow-up. The use of registries is particularly valuable in monitoring a trial's participants for long-term health effects after the trial has ended, since no routine contact with participants is required. Trials should focus on behaviours or activities that have the potential for widespread adoption by groups at risk; these may also vary between nations. For example, the ATBC trial results received much greater attention (and had a correspondingly greater potential effect on individuals' behaviours) in the United States than in Finland, where the trial was conducted. This may reflect a tendency for United States residents to have strong prior beliefs in the efficacy of vitamins or natural foods in protecting against chronic disease, which would make them receptive to interventions involving such nutrients. As this conference has demonstrated, we need scientifically rigorous rationales for trials, and we need a lot more experience with the design and conduct of large-scale trials for prevention of cancers.

Acknowledgement

This project is supported by cooperative agreement UO1-CA 34847 from the National Cancer Institute.

References

1 Parkin DM, Pisani P, Ferlay J. Estimates of the worldwide incidence of eighteen major cancers in 1985. *Int J Cancer*, 1993, 54:594–606.

2 Pisani P, Parkin DM, Ferlay J. Estimates of the worldwide mortality from eighteen major cancers in 1985, Implications for prevention and projections of future burden. *Int J Cancer*, 1993, 55:891–903.

3 Boring CC et al. Cancer statistics 1994, CA: A. *Cancer J Clin*, 1994, 44:7–26.

4 Roemer R. *Legislative Action to Combat the World Tobacco Epidemic*, 2nd edn. Geneva, World Health Organization, 1993.

5 Hammond EC, Horn D. Smoking and death rates: report on forty-four months of 187,783 men. Section II: Death rates by cause. *JAMA*, 1958, 166:1294–1308.

6 Doll R, Hill AB. Lung cancer and other causes of death in relation to smoking: second report on mortality of British doctors. *Br Med J*, 1956, 2:1071–1081.

7 Centers for Disease Control. Cigarette smoking among adults – United States, 1992. *MMWR*, 1994, 43:342–346.

8 Schoenborn CA, Boyd GM. Smoking and other tobacco use: United States, 1987. *Vital Health Stat*, 1989, 10:17.

9 Hammond EC, Selikoff IJ, Seidman H. Asbestos exposure, cigarette smoking and death rates. *Ann NY Acad Sci*, 1979, 330:473–490.

10 Doll R, Peto J. *Effects on Health of Exposure to Asbestos*. London, HMSO, 1985.

11 Nicholson WJ, Perkel G, Selikoff IJ. Occupational exposure to asbestos: population at risk and projected mortality: 1980–2030. *Amer J Ind Med*, 1982, 3:259–311.

12 Omenn GS et al. Contribution of environmental fibers to respiratory cancer. *Env Health Perspect*, 1986, 70:51–56.

13 Peto R et al. Can dietary beta-carotene materially reduce human cancer rates? *Nature*, 1981, 290:201–209.

14 Malone WF. Studies evaluating antioxidants and beta-carotene as chemopreventives. *Am J Clin Nutr*, 1991, 53, 305S–313S.

15 van Poppel G. Carotenoids and cancer: an update with emphasis on human intervention studies. *Eur J Cancer*, 1993, 29A/9:1335–1344.

16 Stich HF et al. Remission of oral leukoplakias and micronuclei in tobacco/betel quid chewers treated with beta-carotene and with beta-carotene plus vitamin A. *Int J Cancer*, 1988, 42:195–199.

17 van Poppel G, Kok FJ, Hermus RJ. Beta-carotene supplementation in smokers reduces the frequency of micronuclei in sputum. *Br J Cancer*, 1992, 66:164–168.

18 Hong WK et al. Prevention of second primary tumors with isotretinoin in squamous-cell carcinoma of the head and neck. *N Engl J Med*, 1990, 323:795–801.

19 Pastorino U et al. Lung cancer chemoprevention. In: Pastorino U, Hong WK, eds. *Chemoimmuno Prevention of Cancer*. New York/Stuttgart, Thiemes Medical Publishers, 1991:147–159.

20 Moon TE et al. and the Arizona Skin Cancer Study Group. Chemoprevention and etiology of non-melanoma skin cancers. *Abstract, Proceedings of the 17th Annual Meeting of the American Society of Preventive Oncology, Tuscon, AZ, USA*, 1993.

21 Greenberg ER et al. A clinical trial of beta carotene to prevent basal-cell and squamous-cell cancers of the skin. The Skin Cancer Prevention Study Group. *N Engl J Med*, 1990, 323:789–95.

22 Tangrea JA et al. and other members of the Isotretinoin-Basal Cell Carcinoma Study Group. Long-term therapy with low-dose isotretinoin for prevention of basal cell carcinoma: a multicenter clinical trial. *J Natl Cancer Inst*, 1992, 84:328–332.

23 Arnold AM et al. The effect of synthetic retinoid etretinate on sputum cytology: results from a randomized trial. *Br J Cancer*, 1992, 65:737–743.

24 McLarty JW. Beta-carotene, vitamin A and lung cancer chemoprevention: results of an intermediate endpoint study. *Am J Clin Nutr*, 1995, 62:1431S.

25 Lee IS et al. A randomized placebo-controlled chemoprevention trial of 13-cis-retinoic acid (cRA) in bronchial squamous metaplasia. *Proc Ann Mtg Amer Soc Clin Oncol*, 1993, 12:335.

26 Goss GD, McBurney MW. Physiological and clinical aspects of vitamin A and its metabolites. *Critical Reviews in Clin Lab Sci*, 1992, 29:185–215.

27 Prabhala RH et al. The effects of 13-cis-retinoic acid and beta-carotene on cellular immunity in humans. *Cancer*, 1991, 67:1556–1560.

28 Hennekens CH, Eberlein K. A randomized trial of aspirin and beta-carotene among US physicians. *Prev Med*, 1985, 14:165–168.

29 The Alpha-Tocopherol, Beta-Carotene Cancer Prevention Study Group. The effect of vitamin E and beta carotene on the incidence of lung cancer and other cancers in male smokers. *New Engl J Med*, 1994, 330:1029–1035.

30 Thornquist MD et al. Statistical design and monitoring of the Carotene and Retinol Efficacy Trial (CARET). *Controlled Clin Trials*, 1993, 14:308–324.

31 Omenn GS et al. The β-Carotene and Retinol Efficacy Trial (CARET) for chemoprevention of lung cancer in high risk populations: smokers and asbestos-exposed workers. *Cancer Res*, 1994, 54, 2038s–2043s.

32 Goodman GE et al. The Carotene and Retinol Efficacy Trial (CARET) to prevent lung cancer in high-risk populations: pilot study with cigarette smokers. *Cancer Epidemiol Biomarkers Prev*, 1993, 2:389–396.

33 Omenn GS et al. The Carotene and Retinol Efficacy Trial (CARET) to prevent lung cancer in high-risk populations: pilot study with asbestos-exposed workers. *Cancer Epidemiol Biomarkers Prev*, 1993, 2:381–387.

34 US Public Health Service. *The Health Consequences of Involuntary Smoking A Report of the Surgeon General.* US Department of Health and Human Services, Public Health Services, Centers for Disease Control. DHHS Publication No. (CDC), 1986:87–8398.

35 Prentice RL. A case–cohort design for epidemiologic cohort studies and disease prevention trials. *Biometrika*, 1986, 73:1–11.

36 Meinert CL. *Clinical Trials: Design, Conduct and Analysis.* New York, Oxford University Press, 1986.

37 Thornquist MD et al. Maintenance of a chemoprevention trial of lung cancer (CARET) after the conclusion of recruitment (Abstract). In: Rao RS, Deo MG, Sanghui LD, eds. *Proceedings of the XVI International Cancer Congress*, 1994:1181–1185.

38 Pepe MS. Inference for events with dependent risks in multiple endpoint studies. *J Am Stat Assn*, 1991, 86:770–778.

39 Omenn GS et al. Long term vitamin A does not produce clinically-significant hypertriglyceridemia: results from CARET the β-carotene and retinol efficacy trial. *Cancer Epidemiol Biomarkers Prev*, 1994, 3:711–713.

40 Gaziano JM et al. A prospective study of carotenoids in fruits and vegetables and decreased cardiovascular mortality in the elderly. *Annals Epidemiol*, 1995, 5:255–260.

41 Manson JE et al. A secondary prevention trial of antioxidant vitamins and cardiovascular disease in women: rationale, design and methods. *Annals Epidemiol*, 1995, 5:261–269.

42 Sperduto RD et al. The Linxian cataract studies: two nutrition intervention trials. *Arch Ophthalmol*, 1993, 111:1246–1253.

43 Goodman GE, Metch BJ, Omenn GS. The effect of long-term beta-carotene and retinol administration on the serum concentrations of alpha-tocopherol. *Cancer Epidemiol Biomarkers Prev*, 1994, 3:429–432.

44 Omenn GS. What accounts for the association of vegetables and fruits with lower incidence of cancers and coronary heart disease? *Annals Epidemiol*, 1995, 5:333–335.

45 Grizzle J et al. Design of the beta-Carotene and Retinol Efficacy Trial (CARET) for chemoprevention of cancer in populations at high risk: heavy smokers and asbestos-exposed workers. In: Pastorino U, Hong WK, eds. *Chemoimmuno Prevention of Cancer.* New York, Stuttgart-Thiemes Medical Publishers, 1991:167–176.

46 Cullen MR, Merrill WW. The relationship between acute inflammatory cells in lavage fluid and bronchial metaplasia. *Chest*, 1992, 102:688–93.

47 Redlich CA et al. Vitamin A chemoprevention of lung cancer: A short-term biomarker study, *Adv Exp Med Biol*, 1995, 375:17–29.

48 Women's Health Study Research Group. The Women's Health Study: Summary of the study design; Rationale and background. *J Myocardial Ischemia*, 1992, 4:27–40.

49 Blumberg J, Block G. The alpha-tocopherol beta-carotene cancer prevention study in Finland. *Nutrition Rev*, 1994, 52:242–250.

50 Hermanson B et al. Beneficial six-year outcomes of smoking cessation in older men and women with coronary artery disease: results from the CASS registry. *New Engl J Med*, 1988, 319:1365–1369.

51 Stampfer MJ et al. Vitamin E consumption and the risk of coronary disease in women. *New Engl J Med*, 1993, 328:1450–1456.

52 Hennekens CH, Buring JE, Peto R. Antioxidant vitamins – benefits not yet proved. *New Engl J Med*, 1994, 330:1080–1081.

53 Steinmetz KA, Potter JD. Vegetables, fruit and cancer. I. Epidemiology; II. Mechanisms. *Cancer Causes, Control*, 1991, 2:325–357, 427–442.

54 Wattenberg LK et al., eds. *Cancer Chemoprevention*. Boca Raton FL, CRC Press, 1992.

55 Kelloff GJ et al. Chemopreventive drug development: perspectives and progress. *Cancer Epidemiol Biomarkers Prev*, 1994, 3:85–98.

56 Kelloff GJ et al. Approaches to the development and marketing approval of drugs that prevent cancer. *Cancer Epidemiol Biomarkers Prev*, 1995, 4:1–10.

57 Heyman RA. Receptor-selective retinoids and the control of differentiation and apoptosis. *Abstract: Cancer Chemopreventive Agents: Drug Development Status and Future Prospects Conference, Princeton, NJ, USA*. 1994.

58 van Zandwijk N et al. Euroscan: The European organization for research and treatment of cancer (EORTC): Chemoprevention study in lung cancer. *Lung Cancer*, 1993, 9:351–356.

59 Kelloff GJ et al. Strategy and planning for chemopreventive drug development: Clinical development plans I. *J Cell Biochem*, 1994, S20:55–62.

60 Moon RC et al. Chemoprevention of respiratory tract neoplasia in the hamster by oltipraz, alone and in combination. *Int J Oncol*, 1994, 4:661–667.

61 *Cancer Chemopreventive Agents: Drug Development Status and Future Prospects. J Cell Biochem*, 1994, Suppl. 20.

G.S. Omenn, G. Goodman, M. Thornquist and S. Barnhart
Fred Hutchinson Cancer Research Center, Cancer Prevention Research Unit, and the University of Washington Schools of Public Health and of Medicine, Seattle, WA 98195, USA

J. Balmes and D. Liu
Department of Medicine, University of California, San Francisco, CA 94110, USA

M. Cherniack and M. Cullen
Department of Medicine, Yale University, New Haven, CT 06510, USA

A. Glass and B. Valanis
Kaiser Permanente Center for Health Research, Portland, OR 97227, USA

J. Keogh
Department of Medicine, University of Maryland, Baltimore, MD 21201, USA

F. Meyskens, Jr and J. Williams Jr
Department of Medicine and Cancer Center, University of California, Irvine, Orange, CA 92668, USA

M. Perloff
National Cancer Institute, Bethesda, MD, USA

Chemoprevention of breast cancer with fenretinide

U. Veronesi*, G. De Palo, A. Costa, F. Formelli and A. Decensi

Since their discovery, retinoids (analogues of vitamin A) have been known to play an important role in tissue differentiation. In fact, retinoid deficiency is associated with the failure of stem cells to mature into differentiated cells. Retinoids may be able to suppress tumour promotion and to modify some properties of transformed malignant cells, probably by activating and/or repressing specific genes. However, their poor tolerability in humans has limited their use to a few medical indications only, mainly in dermatology. Vitamin A is so greatly involved in a number of different biological processes that its long-term intake can lead to a variety of side-effects and unfavourable events: most of them are reversible and usually disappear rapidly after drug withdrawal (1). A great deal of effort has been put into identifying new synthetic analogues of vitamin A, in order to identify molecules with reduced systemic toxicity (2). Drug tolerability is a major issue in cancer chemoprevention, for the obvious reason that what may be an acceptable toxicity to fight an established disease cannot be considered suitable for merely reducing the probability of developing it.

The important results obtained with isotretinoin in reducing the risk of second primary tumours in the aerodigestive tract in patients previously treated for carcinoma pointed to the need for less toxic and more effective synthetic analogues of vitamin A (3). In fact, one-third of the patients receiving isotretinoin did not complete the 12-month course of treatment because of toxicity or non-compliance (3).

Tolerability of retinoids

The side-effects associated with retinoids, both natural and synthetic, involve different organs (4, 5). Dermatological side-effects may include mucocutaneous dryness and skin atrophy (6). Abnormal skin photosensitivity has also been reported for some vitamin A synthetic analogues (7), and nail dystrophy has also been described (8).

In the case of the eye, retinoids may interfere with some of the mechanisms of vision, in particular

*Correspondence: U. Veronesi, European Institute of Oncology, Via Ripamonti 435, 20141 Milan, Italy.

dark adaptation (9). Vision is activated in the following way: in the rod outer segment of the retina, rhodopsin is catalysed into opsin and retinal by light; this reaction leads to the generation of the nervous impulse which goes to the brain. Since retinal is converted from retinol, a sufficient amount of the latter must always be available in the retina to guarantee its proper functioning (10).

Retinoid-induced skeletal changes in humans as a result of both hypervitaminosis A and retinoid therapy have been reported during the last 40 years; these changes have manifested mainly as hyperostosis (11).

Increases in triglyceride, cholesterol and HDL cholesterol are uncommon in patients treated with synthetic retinoids (12). Bershad et al. (13) reported changes in plasma lipids during isotretinoin therapy for acne. Lipid abnormalities included elevated triglycerides, decreased HDL and increased cholesterol; the LDL/HDL cholesterol ratio showed a significant but reversible increase.

With regard to teratogenicity, the spectrum of congenital defects induced by synthetic retinoids seems to be identical to that induced by retinoic acid when it develops an embryopathic action (14).

Retinoids in differentiation, proliferation and carcinogenesis

In their study on the effects of retinoid deficiency in the rat, Wolbach & Howe (15) demonstrated the important effects of retinoids on both cellular differentiation and proliferation, and indicated that retinoids would be significant molecules in the study of carcinogenesis. They clearly recognized that retinoid deficiency was accompanied by enhanced cellular proliferation, with the formation of lesions resembling those in malignant or premalignant conditions.

It was later shown that retinoids are required to maintain normal differentiation in most cells in the mammalian organs, during both embryogenesis and adult life (16). As some three-quarters of all primary cancers in both men and women derive from epithelial tissues that depend on retinoids for appropriate cell differentiation, research into the role of

Table 1. Reversible impaired dark adaptation confirmed by abnormal electroretinograms in patients treated with 4-HPR

Dose (mg/day)	Treatment period	No. of patients with impaired dark adaptation/total	Source
800	2 weeks	2/5	Kaiser-Kupfer (32)
600	3 weeks	2/8	Kingstone (33)
400	1–2 months	1/31	Modiano (34)
300	6 months	1/25	Costa (31)

retinoids in carcinogenesis appears essential. Sporn et al. (16) developed a tracheal organ culture system to study the relationship between the molecular structure and cellular activity of hundreds of natural and synthetic retinoids (17, 18). In the absence of retinoids, the tracheal epithelium loses its normal, columnar, ciliated and mucous cells, and develops proliferative lesions characterized by heavy squamous metaplasia. The addition of retinoids to the tracheal organ cultures results in the reversal of keratinization, the reappearance of normal, ciliated and mucous cells, and the suppression of the excessive proliferation of basal cells. Since retinoids exert such control over cell differentiation and cell proliferation, it is clearly important to investigate whether they might be useful agents in the prevention of carcinogenesis *in vivo*. This approach involves an enhancement of the intrinsic physiological mechanisms that protect against the development of mutant clones. Since the process of carcinogenesis is partly characterized by loss of cellular differentiation and growth control, and since retinoids both inhibit growth and induce or enhance cellular differentiation, their use in an attempt to arrest or reverse the process of carcinogenesis represents a physiological approach.

Data providing a better understanding of the mechanisms involved in the action of retinoids are becoming available from the laboratory (19). A great deal is known about nuclear retinoic acid receptors (RARs), which may be the mediators of the inhibition of carcinogenesis induced by both natural and synthetic retinoids (20, 21). Another important activity of retinoids is their ability to induce apoptosis in human neoplastic cells (22, 23).

The synthetic retinoid fenretinide (4-HPR)

In order to obtain greater efficacy and fewer side-effects, more than 1000 different retinoids have

been synthesized in the last 30 years by modifying the ring structure, the side chain or the terminal group of the molecule. An interesting vitamin A analogue presently being studied for breast cancer chemoprevention is the synthetic retinoid N-(4-hydroxyphenyl)-retinamide (4-HPR; fenretinide) (24). Fenretinide was synthesized in the United States in the late 1960s, and its biological activity was assayed by Sporn & Newton (25) who showed the tendency of this compound to accumulate in the breast instead of the liver. The inhibition by 4-HPR of chemically induced mammary carcinoma in rats was described by Moon et al. (26). Fenretinide has since been studied extensively and has been proved to be non-genotoxic and less toxic than many other retinoids (27). On the basis of these data, 4-HPR has been proposed for chemopreventive evaluation in human breast cancer.

Pharmacological studies

Studies on the pharmacokinetics of 4-HPR have been conducted in breast cancer patients who participated in a phase I trial and continued to be treated and monitored for 5 years (28, 29). Before the large randomized trial, a series of planned studies were carried out. The plasma concentrations of 4-HPR, its main metabolite 4-MPR (4-methoxyphenyl-retinamide), and retinol were measured by high-performance liquid chromatography (28) after different doses and at different times during and after treatment.

During the phase I study, it was shown that, as previously reported in rats (30), 4-HPR causes an early reduction of plasma retinol concentrations in humans (28). Twenty-four hours after a single dose of 200 mg, the concentrations of retinol and its specific transport protein, retinol-binding protein (RBP), were reduced in all the treated patients, with average reductions of 38% and 26%, respectively. The reduction of plasma retinol concentration was proportional to the dose, and it was associated with impaired dark adaptation, a side-effect reported in patients treated with 4-HPR (9, 31, 32, 33, 34). As shown in Table 1, this side-effect occurred at different rates according to the tested dose. In order to minimize this side-effect, it was decided periodically to interrupt drug treatment, on a temporary basis, so as to increase plasma retinol concentrations, thus allowing storage of retinol in the retina. A 3-day interruption in treatment at the end of each month was prescribed to the patients of the ongoing trial.

The reduction of plasma retinol levels has been shown to be associated with the interaction between 4-HPR and RBP (the specific transport protein of retinol in plasma), and with interference with the RBP-transthyretin complex formation (35).

Daily administration of 200 mg of 4-HPR results in average 4-HPR concentrations of 350 ng/ml 12 hours after drug intake, i.e. approximately 1 μM (Fig. 1), and these are constant throughout the treatment period. The concentrations of 4-MPR, which are similar to those of the parent drug, increase slightly but significantly during the first 34 months of treatment, but after 5 years, they are similar to those found at 5 months. Retinol concentrations are reduced from 493 to approximately 170 ng/ml (i.e. by 65%), and this reduction is constant during the 5-year treatment.

After 5 years of treatment, 4-HPR was cleared from plasma with an average $t^{1/2}\beta$ of 27 hours, as evaluated using blood collected from 14 patients between 12 and 86 hours after the last drug intake (Table 2). The rate of elimination of 4-MPR was lower than that of the parent drug, with an average $t^{1/2}\beta$ of 54 hours. A comparison between retinol

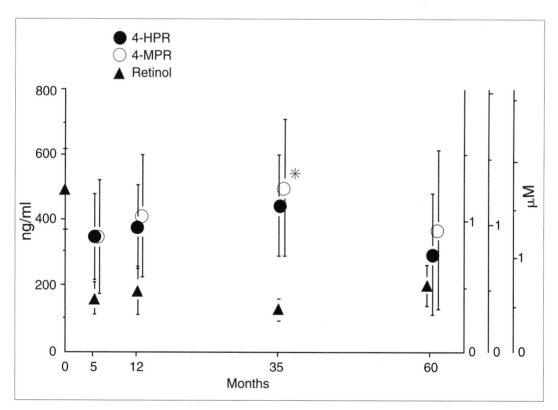

Fig. 1. Plasma concentration of 4-HPR, 4-MPR and retinol during 5-year chronic treatment. Plasma was collected from seven patients about 14 hours (range 12–19) after the last drug intake, at 5, 12, 35 and 60 months after the beginning of treatment. Baseline retinol concentrations are also reported. Points, means; bars, SD. *$p < 0.05$ by Dunnet's t-test versus 5 months (redrawn from 23).

Table 2. Regression coefficients (b) and $t^{1/2}$ β (mean ± SD) after 5-year 4-HPR treatment at 200 mg/day[a]			
Substance	**b**	**c.v.[b] (%)**	**$t^{1/2}$ β (hours)**
4-HPR	− 0.032 93 ± 0.004 34	13	27 ± 4.41
4-MPR	− 0.013 62 ± 0.003 36	25	54 ± 13.92
Retinol	+ 0.012 78 ± 0.002 53	20	

[a]After 5 years treatment, blood was taken from 14 patients at three different times in the 12–85 hours after the last drug intake.
[b]c.v., coefficient of variation (from 23).

and 4-HPR average b values indicated that, in the period of time examined, the ratio between the rate of 4-HPR elimination ($b = − 0.032\,93$) and the rate of retinol recovery ($b = + 0.012\,78$) was 2.58.

Distribution of 4-HPR in the breast

Breast biopsies in a small sample of patients confirmed the ability of this retinoid to accumulate in the breast, as already demonstrated in rodents (26) and as previously reported in other breast cancer patients (36). The concentrations of 4-HPR were 1.4–8.2 times those in plasma. 4-MPR, which is more lipophilic than the parent drug, accumulated in the breast to an even greater extent. This might be relevant to the chemopreventive effect of this retinoid, since this metabolite has the same potency as 4-HPR in *in vitro* differentiation assays (37). In fact, this retinoid accumulates not only in fat but also in the epithelial cells of the breast, as shown by the concentrations of 4-HPR and 4-MPR in the nipple

Table 3. 4-HPR and 4-MPR concentrations (ng/ml) in plasma and nipple discharge[a]				
	4-HPR	**R[b]**	**4-MPR**	**R**
Plasma	212		240	
Nipple discharge				
Right breast	2900	14	5740	24
Left breast	2600	12	8220	34

[a]4-HPR (200 mg/day) was administered for 15 days. Blood and nipple discharge were collected 22 hours after the last dose.
[b]R, nipple concentrations/plasma concentrations (from 23).

discharge, which were 10 and 30 times higher, respectively, than those found in plasma (Table 3).

Fenretinide breast cancer chemoprevention study

The original idea of studying this retinoid in a population of early stage breast cancer patients was developed by us in the early 1980s (38). The concept was that patients treated for an early cancer with a good prognosis have a known risk of developing an independent contralateral breast carcinoma. The main advantage of this model is that the incidence of contralateral breast cancer is well assessed, i.e. about 0.8% per year, and that this figure is fairly stable after surgery in patients who have experienced a primary cancer in the breast. Moreover, as these patients are already under medical control with periodic follow-up, participation in the study for the required long period of time is easier, and compliance is expected to be higher than in the general population.

The first protocol of a randomized clinical trial to evaluate the efficacy of 4-HPR in preventing contralateral breast cancer was designed in 1984. The study was awarded an NCI grant in 1985 but was put on hold a few months later as a result of toxicity data arising from other sources who were using doses of 600 mg/day. With the aim of verifying a possible relationship between the dose and the reported side-effects (night blindness and erythema; 31, 39), a phase I study was started in January 1986, which led us to identify the best-tolerated dose (200 mg/day with a 3-day interruption in treatment at the end of each month).

Recruitment of patients for the phase III randomized study began in March 1987. The final objective of the study is obvious. If fenretinide were successful in preventing second primaries in breast

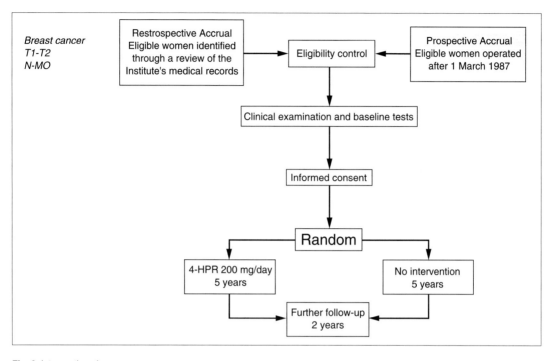

Fig. 2. Intervention plan.

cancer patients, it would possibly be effective for wider groups of subjects at high risk of breast cancer in the general population. Study participants were breast cancer patients aged 30–70 years who had been treated with ablative or conservative (plus RT) surgery for a T1 tumour (< 2 cm) or a T2 tumour (< 5 cm), without nodal metastases. Infiltrating carcinomas of all histological types were eligible, as was ductal carcinoma-*in-situ*. In order to be eligible, patients had to show no evidence of local recurrences and/or distant metastases, they had to have had no previous treatment with adjuvant chemotherapy and/or hormone therapy, and the results of their metabolic and liver function tests had to be normal. Patients had to declare that they would not have children during the study. The following were excluded: patients with previous neoplastic disease (with the exception of basal cell carcinoma of the skin and CIN); patients with lobular *in situ* carcinoma or Paget's disease; patients who lived in a remote, inaccessible region; patients with neuropsychiatric difficulties; patients with ocular diseases; and patients who were participating in another study. Patients entered the study through

one of two routes: those who were identified as potentially eligible through a review of the medical records, and those who had been operated on after 1 March 1987 and proved to be eligible (Fig. 2).

At baseline the following tests were performed: general and dermatologic examination, laboratory tests (HB, HT, WBC, PLTS, SGOT, SGPT, BIL, AP, total proteins, BUN, creatinine, blood sugar, cholesterol, triglycerides, retinol blood levels), a pregnancy test (for those at a fertile age), mammography, chest X-ray, bone scan and liver echography. An ocular questionnaire was also filled out by the patient. It was designed by us according to the areas likely to be affected by fenretinide administration: dark adaptation, vision in conditions of poor luminosity, recovery after dazzling. The ocular questionnaire was considered positive if at least two out of the three items were positive, and doubtful if one out of the three was positive. If the results of this test proved negative the subject was considered eligible. The ocular questionnaire was performed at every control. Both groups, intervention and control, underwent the same tests in follow-up. The follow-up schedule consisted of a physical examination and

Table 4. 4-HPR breast cancer study (total cases at closure of recruitment 31 July 1993)			
	4-HPR	**CTR**	**Total**
Randomized	1496 (50.3%)	1476 (49.7%)	2972
Early refusal	−23 (0.8%)	−3 (0.1%)	−26
Protocol violation	−37 (1.2%)	−32 (1.1%)	−69
Early lost	−15 (0.5%)	−14(0.5%)	−29
Evaluable	**1421 (47.8%)**	**1427 (48%)**	**2848**
Pre-menopause	660 (48.2%)	710 (51.8%)	1370
Post-menopause	761 (51.5%)	717 (48.5%)	1478
Conservative treatment	899 (50.1%)	896 (49.9%)	1795
Ablative treatment	522 (49.6%)	531 (50.4%)	1053

laboratory tests every 6 months, a mammography, chest X-ray and liver echography every year, a bone scan at 18, 36 and 60 months, and measurements of 4-HPR and retinol levels each year in all treated patients.

The patient's compliance is assessed according to four elements: physician's confidence in the patient; pill count; plasma assay of 4-HPR and its principal metabolite 4-MPR and number of visits. Before joining the study, each patient was counselled by the investigating physician on the aims of the study, the expected drug effects, and the side-effects. It was explained to the patient that it is important to take the drug daily, both capsules after dinner, to increase the bioavailability of 4-HPR.

The sample size was calculated as follows: assuming that a 3-year lag time is required to obtain full intervention efficacy and taking into account a 2-year follow-up of all patients after the end of intervention, the required sample size was 3500 subjects for an expected 50% reduction in the incidence rate of contralateral breast cancer, with a drop-out of 10% (38).

Recruitment was closed on 31 July 1993 with a total of 2972 patients (Table 4). The study was closed because of a considerable reduction in the recruitment rate, due to the widespread dissemination of the NCI Medical Alert recommending 'some form of adjuvant treatments' in all patients treated with breast cancers (with positive and negative axillary nodes), and to the growing evidence that tamoxifen might reduce the incidence of contralateral new primaries in breast cancer patients.

Entry criteria violations were found in 69 patients (2.3%). Twenty-six patients (0.9%) refused to enter the study after having signed the informed consent form and 29 patients (1%) were lost at follow-up. The total number of evaluable cases was 2848 (1421 in the 4-HPR group and 1427 in the control group). The two groups were well balanced for menopausal status, primary tumour treatment, histology and tumour size. In 49% of the cases, the time that had elapsed between surgery and randomization was less than 1 year, and in 31.5% of the cases it was between 1 and 3 years. Out of 2848 evaluable patients, 867 completed the first 5 years, 1141 are still ongoing, and a total of 840 patients have interrupted the study for various reasons, mainly because of the occurrence of neoplastic events (loco-regional relapses, distant relapses, contralateral carcinomas or new primaries). The results of the study will be available in 2 years.

References

1 Yob EH, Pochi PE. Side effects and long-term toxicity of synthetic retinoids. *Arch Dermatol*, 1987, 123:1375–1378.

2 Moon RC, Mehta RG. Chemoprevention of experimental carcinogenesis in animals. *Prev Med*, 1989, 18:576–591.

3 Hong WK et al. Prevention of second primary tumors with isotretinoin in squamous-cell carcinoma of the head and neck. *N Engl J Med*, 1990, 323:795–801.

4 Smith MA et al. Retinoids in cancer therapy. *J Clin Oncol*, 1992, 10:839–864.

5 Warrell PR, Jr, Pastorino U, Decensi A. Clinical Toxicology of the Retinoids. In: Degos L, Parkinson DR, eds. *Retinoids in Oncology*. ESO Monographs Springer, 1995:67–71.

6 Hoting E, Meissner K. Arotinoid-ethylester, effectiveness in refractory cutaneous T-cell lymphoma. *Cancer*, 1988, 62:1044–1048.

7 Ferguson J, Johnson BE. Retinoid associated phototoxicity and photosensitivity. *Pharmacol Ther*, 1989, 40:123–125.

8 Ferguson J, Simpson NB, Hammersley N. Severe nail distrophy associated with retinoid therapy. *Lancet*, 1983, 2:974.

9 Decensi A et al. Effect of the synthetic retinoid fenretinide on dark adaptation and the ocular surface. *J Natl Cancer Inst*, 1994, 86:1105–1110.

10 Pawson BA. A historical introduction to the chemistry of vitamin A and its analogues (retinoids). *Ann NY Acad Sci*, 1981, 359:1–8.

11 Kilcoyne RF. Effect of retinoids on bone. *J Am Acad Dermatol*, 1988, 19:212–216.

12 Marsden JR. Lipid metabolism and retinoid therapy. *Pharmacol Ther*, 1989, 40:55–65

13 Bershad S et al. Changes in plasma lipids and lipoproteins during isotretinoin therapy for acne. *N Engl J Med*, 1985, 313: 981–985.

14 Flanagan JL, Wilhite CC, Ferm VH. Comparative teratogenic activity of cancer chemopreventive retinoidal benzoic acid congeners (arotinoids). *J Natl Cancer Inst*, 1987, 78:533–538.

15 Wolbach SB, Howe PR. Tissue changes following deprivation of fat soluble A vitamin. *J Exp Med*, 1925, 42:753–777.

16 Sporn MB et al. Prevention of chemical carcinogenesis by vitamin A and its synthetic analogs (retinoids). *Fed Proc*, 1976, 35:1332–1338.

17 Sporn MB et al. Relationships between structure and activity of retinoids. *Nature*, 1976, 263:110–113.

18 Newton DL, Henderson WR, Sporn MB. Structure activity relationships of retinoids in hamster tracheal organ culture. *Cancer Res*, 1980, 40:3413–3425.

19 Hong WK et al. Retinoid chemoprevention of aerodigestive cancer: from basic research to the clinic. *Clin Cancer Res*, 1995, 1: 677–686.

20 Xu XC et al. Differential expression of nuclear retinoic acid receptors in normal, premalignant, and malignant head and neck tissues. *Cancer Res*, 1994, 54: 3580–5387.

21 Lotan R et al. Suppression of retinoic acid receptor β in premalignant oral lesions and its upregulation by isotretinoin. *N Engl J Med*, 1995, 332: 1405–1410.

22 Delia D et al. N-(4-hydroxyphenyl)retinamide induces apoptosis of malignant hematopoietic cell lines including those unresponsive to retinoic acid. *Cancer Res*, 1993, 53:6063–6041.

23 Ponzoni M et al. Differential effects of N-(4-Hydroxyphenyl)retinamide and retinoic acid on neuroblastoma cells: apoptosis versus differentiation. *Cancer Res*, 1995, 55:853–861.

24 Costa A. Biological approaches to breast cancer prevention. *The Breast*, 1992, 1:119–123.

25 Sporn MB, Newton DL. Chemoprevention of cancer with retinoids. *Fed Proc*, 1979, 38:2528–2534.

26 Moon RC et al. N-(4-hydroxyphenyl) retinamide, a new retinoid for prevention of breast cancer. *Cancer Res*, 1979, 39:1339–1346.

27 Paulson JD et al. Lack of genotoxicity of the cancer chemopreventive agent N-(4-hydroxyphenyl) retinamide. *Fund Appl Toxicol*, 1995, 5:144–150.

28 Formelli F et al. Plasma retinol level reduction by the synthetic retinoid fenretinide: a one year follow-up study of breast cancer patients. *Cancer Res*, 1989, 49: 6149–6152.

29 Formelli F et al. Five-year administration of fenretinide: pharmacokinetics and effects on plasma retinol concentrations. *J Clin Oncol*, 1993, 11: 2036–2042.

30 Formelli F, Carsana R, Costa A. N-(4-Hydroxyphenyl)retinamide (4-HPR) lowers plasma retinol levels in rats. *Med Sci Res*, 1987, 15:843–844.

31 Costa A et al. Tolerability of the synthetic retinoid fenretinide (HPR). *Eur J Cancer Clin Oncol*, 1989, 25:805–809.

32 Kaiser-Kupfer MI, Peck GL, Caruso RC. Abnormal retinal function associated with fenretinide, a synthetic retinoid. *Arch Ophthalmol*, 1986, 104:69–70.

33 Kingstone TP et al. Visual cutaneous toxicity which occurs during N-(4-hydroxyphenyl) retinamide therapy for psoriasis. *Clin Exp Dermatol*, 1986, 11:624–627.

34 Modiano MR et al. Ocular toxic effects of Fenretinide. *J Natl Cancer Inst*, 1990, 82:1063.

35 Berni R, Formelli F. In vitro interaction of fenretinide with plasma retinol-binding protein and its functional consequences. *FEBS Lett*, 1992, 308:43–45.

36 Metha RG et al. Distribution of fenretinide in the mammary gland of breast cancer patients. *Eur J Cancer*, 1991, 27:138–141.
37 Swanson BN et al. Biotransformation and biological activity of N(4-hydroxyphenyl)retinamide derivatives in rodents. *J Pharmacol Exp Ther*, 1981, 219:632–637.
38 Veronesi U et al. Chemoprevention of breast cancer with retinoids. *NCI Monographs*, 1992, 12:93–97.
39 Rotmensz N et al. Long term tolerability of fenretinide (4-HPR) in breast cancer patients. *Eur J Cancer*, 1991, 2:1127–1131.

U. Veronesi and A. Costa
European Institute of Oncology, Via Ripamonti 435, 20141 Milan, Italy

G. De Palo and F. Formelli
Istituto Nazionale Tumori, Via G. Venezian 1, 20133 Milan, Italy

A. Decensi
FIRC Chemoprevention Research Unit, Milan/Genoa, Italy

Chemoprevention of breast cancer with tamoxifen

J. Cuzick

Breast cancer is the most common cancer in women worldwide, affecting both the developing and developed worlds. Over 750 000 cases (1) and 300 000 deaths (2) occur each year. Although there are a large number of empirical risk factors, very little is understood about the specific agents or mechanisms that cause breast cancer, and this makes primary prevention very difficult. The rapid increases in the incidence of the disease now occurring in developing countries and the dramatic change among Japanese migrants to the United States, in whom rates approximate those of the white population by the second generation, strongly favour the argument that, on a population basis, the major risk factors are due to lifestyle and environmental factors. However, within populations, there is a clear tendency for the disease to run in families. The risk of breast cancer is approximately doubled if a woman's mother or sister developed breast cancer by the age of 50 and is much higher (approximately 10-fold) if her mother or sister developed bilateral cancer before the age of 40. Some of this familial tendency is due to rare dominant genes (BRCA1 and BRCA2) with very high penetrance, but most familial cancer is probably due to less penetrant 'susceptibility genes' in which environmental and lifestyle factors are also important.

Although the details are poorly understood, there is considerable evidence and agreement that both environmental and genetic factors exert their influence by a hormonal mechanism, and that the sex steroids play a crucial role in breast carcinogenesis. Two suggested approaches to breast cancer prevention, i.e. dietary fat restriction and increased amounts of exercise, may actually exert their protective effect by influencing hormonal levels and balances. However, both of these approaches have very major logistic obstacles which hinder their scientific evaluation. In the case of dietary fat restriction, we still do not have a clear indication of which types of fat are likely to be bad, and to achieve a blanket reduction of all fat intake that is of a large enough magnitude to be effective over a prolonged period is likely to be very difficult. Furthermore, some of the evidence from migrant studies and other sources indirectly suggests that it may be diet during adolescence which determines hormonal profiles (3), and thus it would take 40 years before any significant effect on breast cancer became apparent. A similar problem relates to any prospective study of the effect of regular exercise, where once again the data to date suggest that the adolescent period may be the most important one for determining risks. Such trials are only feasible if reliable intermediate end-points are found which can be evaluated many years earlier.

A more direct approach to breast cancer prevention is to attempt to devise an oral contraceptive that reduces the risk of breast cancer. Current combined oral contraceptives reduce the risk of ovarian and endometrial cancers, and Pike and colleagues (4) have pioneered the use of an LHRH-agonist (7.5 mg leuprolide acetate as a depot every 28 days), coupled with adding back small amounts of oestradiol and androgen and infrequent courses of a progestagen, as a chemopreventive strategy in younger women.

For logistic reasons, it is highly desirable to study interventions that affect the late stages of carcinogenesis, as opposed to early events, so that any effect can be observed within 10–15 years. For breast cancer, the existence of late-stage factors which can be manipulated is clearly apparent from the fact that age at menopause has a more than threefold effect on the risk of cancer (5).

Of the direct chemopreventive measures, only two have reached the maturity to warrant large-scale clinical trials. The use of retinoids is discussed elsewhere in this book, and here we will focus on the use of the oestrogen agonist tamoxifen.

Why tamoxifen?
Breast cancer reduction

Tamoxifen has long been used to treat breast cancer. It is a triphenylethylene derivative (Fig. 1) with both oestrogenic and anti-oestrogenic properties (6). It was originally designed as an oral contraceptive but was found to increase fertility and thus was shelved for many years. It still has a limited use in treating infertility, but was first used to treat advanced breast cancer in 1969. Response rates

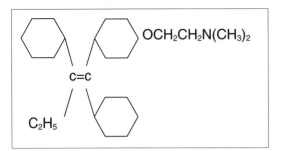

Fig. 1. Chemical structure of tamoxifen.

are about 30% and it is still the first line of treatment for advanced disease in women who have not already received it. Trials of tamoxifen's use in early breast cancer to prevent recurrence began in 1974 and to date over 6 000 000 women-years of experience have accrued. Results on over 30 000

women in randomized trials have been summarized in a detailed overview (7). Fig. 2 shows that overall recurrence rates were reduced by 25% and mortality rates were down by 17%. Most trials used tamoxifen for 2 years. Better results were found in trials that used tamoxifen for more than 2 years, where the reduction in recurrence rates was 38% and the mortality rates were reduced by 24%.

The best evidence for a preventive effect of tamoxifen comes from examining the incidence of new contralateral tumours in women with cancer in one breast who are participating in randomized trials of tamoxifen. An initial report (8) showed a very large early reduction in new tumours in a trial using tamoxifen for 2 years (Fig. 3). Two subsequent (overlapping) overviews (9, 7) have shown an approximately 40% reduction in new tumours. Again, the effects were greater in trials using a longer duration of tamoxifen (26%, 37% and 53%

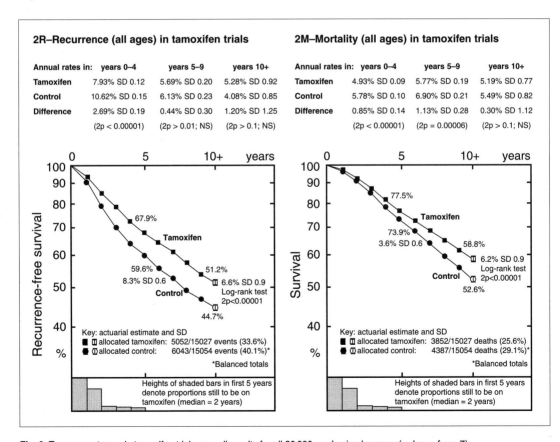

Fig. 2. Ten-year outcome in tamoxifen trials: overall results for all 30 000 randomized women (redrawn from 7).

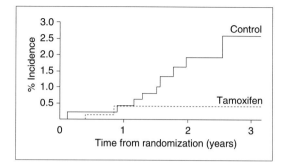

Fig. 3. Cumulative incidence of contralateral breast cancers in patients in an adjuvant trial of two years of tamoxifen (redrawn from *8*).

in trials of less than 2 years, 2 years, and more than 2 years of tamoxifen, respectively). However, further follow-up of the original report cited above has reduced the extent of the benefit associated with tamoxifen, suggesting that long-term treatment (more than 2 years) may be necessary to achieve long-term protection (*10*). This has also been found in animal studies (*11*), where early and prolonged use of tamoxifen has led to greater protection against chemically induced tumours.

The primary mechanism by which tamoxifen is thought to work is through its agonist properties which allow it to bind to the oestrogen receptor and block the effects of the more powerful endogenous oestrogens (*6*). However, several clinical studies have shown that tamoxifen is also effective in women with receptor-negative tumours, and a host of other potential antitumour activities have been described, including the modulation of the expression of growth factors (TGF-β, EGF and IGF-1) and oncogene, and the inhibition of enzymes involved in the synthesis of oestrogens and signal transduction (*12*).

Reduction in cardiovascular disease

Several studies have found that tamoxifen reduces cholesterol levels (Table 1). The effect is greater for the LDL-cholesterol fraction and, overall, a 20 mg daily dose appears to reduce levels by about 15–20%. In most studies the effects on HDL-cholesterol have been small and non-significant, suggesting a substantial benefit for cardiovascular disease. Two clinical trials have now reported evidence to confirm this. In a Scottish trial, deaths from myocardial infarction were reduced by 60%, from 25 cases to 10 cases (*13*). Subsequently, in a Swedish trial, Rutqvist & Mattson (*14*), found that there was a significant 30% reduction in hospital admissions for cardiac disease in women taking tamoxifen, and that the effects were greater after

Study (Ref.)	Menopausal status	No. of subjects	Duration	Total cholesterol (% change)	LDL (% change)	HDL (% change)
Rossner and Wallgren (*77*)	Post	11	2 months	14 (↓)	20 (↓)	9 (↓)
Caleffi et al. (*78*)	Pre	10	3 months	7 (↓)	12 (↓)	11 (↓)
Bruning et al. (*79*)	Pre	4	6 months	7 (↓)	18 (↓)	18 (↑)
	Post	31	6 months	7 (↓)	13 (↓)	8 (↑)
Love et al. (*80*)	Post	65	12 months	12 (↓)	20 (↓)	7 (↓)
Dewar et al. (*81*)	Post	24	5 years	15 (↓)	–	–
Cuzick et al. (*16*)	Post	14/47[a]	~6 years	12 (↓)	22 (↓)	14 (↓)
Love et al. (*15*)	Post	7	3 months	20 (↓)	–	–
Thangaraju et al. (*82*)	Post	39	6 months	15 (↓)	12 (↓)	11 (↑)
Dziewulska-Bokiniec et al. (*83*)	Post	45/33a	6–73 months	16 (↓)	18 (↓)	1 (↑)

Table 1. Studies of the effect of tamoxifen on cholesterol levels in terms of percentage change from baseline (most patients received 20 mg/day)

[a]Untreated patients used as controls in place of baseline measurements.

5 years of treatment than after 2 years. Both of these studies were on post-menopausal women, where the cholesterol levels and rates of cardiovascular disease are much higher. Cardiovascular disease is much rarer in pre-menopausal women and there is little evidence of the effect of tamoxifen on cholesterol levels, and no evidence of its effect on cardiovascular disease, in these women. Love, Mambi & Feyzi (15) have shown that the effects on lipids occur within 2 weeks of tamoxifen administration,

Table 2. Side-effects in the Royal Marsden Pilot Prevention Trial[a] (28)			
	Tamoxifen	**Placebo**	**Significance**
Total number	920	926	
Hormone replacement therapy			
Before randomization	131 (14)	134 (14)	NS
On treatment	126 (14)	119 (13)	NS
Total	257 (28)	253 (27)	NS
Hysterectomy	2 (3)	16 (2)	NS
Ovarian surgery	14 (2)	15 (2)	NS
Side-effects			
Not receiving HRT[b]	507	531	
Nausea	41 (6)	65 (10)	P = 0.02
Non-compliance	16	11	NS
Vomiting	3 (<1)	9 (1)	NS
Headache	82 (12)	96 (14)	NS
Non-compliance	10	19	NS
Hot flushes			
Pre-menopausal	151 (36)	75 (17)	P < 0.001
Post-menopausal	66 (29)	54 (25)	NS
Total	225 (34)	134 (20)	P < 0.001
Non-compliance	43	8	P < 0.001
Weight gain	44 (7)	71 (11)	P = 0.01
Non-compliance	9	6	NS
Menstrual irregularities	93 (14)	57 (9)	P = 0.002
Non-compliace	14	4	
Mood change	15 (3)	13 (3)	NS
Non-compliance	12	6	NS
Vaginal discharge			
Pre-menopausal	53 (13)	12 (3)	P < 0.001
Post-menopausal	53 (24)	17 (8)	P < 0.001
Total	108 (16)	30 (4)	P < 0.001
Non-compliance	9	3	NS

NS, not significant.
[a]Figures are for number of women in each group. Numbers in parentheses show percentage of women affected. Non-compliance figures indicate that the side-effect was severe enough to lead to cessation of treatment and are based on all eligible patients.
[b]This number is the denominator for the side-effects given below.

and Cuzick et al. (16) have shown that the levels return to normal after stopping tamoxifen. However, this does not mean that the benefits will stop, as cardiovascular damage is cumulative and any period of lower cholesterol level may translate into some long-term benefit.

Tamoxifen (and especially its metabolite 4-hydroxytamoxifen) has also been shown to inhibit lipid peroxidation in experimental systems, and this antioxidant activity (which is similar to that of 17β-oestradiol) may be another mechanism by which tamoxifen reduces the risk of cardiovascular disease (17, 18). Thangaraju et al. (19) studied 45 post-menopausal women receiving tamoxifen and found that it decreased the rate of lipid peroxidation and increased serum levels of selenium and vitamins A, C and E.

Bone

There are now several studies showing a beneficial effect of tamoxifen on bone density in post-menopausal women. Most studies show an initial increase in trabecular bone, leading to increased spinal bone density and also to a stabilization of cortical bone mass in the femoral neck, as compared with a steady decline in both sites in untreated post-menopausal control women. These effects are similar to those seen in women undergoing hormone replacement therapy and indicate an oestrogenic effect of tamoxifen on bone in post-menopausal women. In the largest reported study, Love, Mazess & Barden (20) reported a 0.61% annual increase in bone density in the lumbar spine in treated patients and a 1.0% annual decrease in controls; similar results have been reported by others (21, 22, 23, 24). Little is known about the effect of tamoxifen on bone in pre-menopausal women. Two published reports (25, 26) found little overall effect, but a recent abstract of a more detailed study suggested there may be some bone loss (27).

Side-effects and long-term risks
Acute side-effects

Several studies have reported on short-term side-effects of tamoxifen, but few have been placebo-controlled trials and so the results are not always easy to interpret. The most useful information comes from the pilot prevention study at the Royal Marsden Hospital, London, where almost 2 000 high-risk women have been randomized to receive

tamoxifen or placebo (28). Hysterectomy rates were non-significantly higher in the tamoxifen arm (3% versus 1.7%) and there was no difference in the rates of ovarian surgery (1.5% versus 1.6%). Baseline levels of HRT usage were virtually identical in both arms of the study (14%), and the requirements for HRT on treatment were similar in the two arms (14% versus 13%). The most prominent side-effects in women not receiving HRT were menopausal symptoms (Table 2). Hot flushes were twice as common in tamoxifen-treated pre-menopausal women (36% versus 17%), but they were of similar prevalence in post-menopausal women (29% versus 25%). Vaginal discharge was more common in those on tamoxifen, both pre- and post-menopause (16% versus 4% overall), and menstrual irregularities were also slightly more common (14% versus 9%). As 62% of the women in this trial were pre-menopausal, it is possible that some of the menopausal symptoms associated with tamoxifen are due merely to the menopause having been brought forward in time. Longer follow-up will be required to see if they converge as more women pass through the menopause. There were no differences in the reported occurrence of headaches, and interestingly, nausea and vomiting, side-effects that have been attributed to tamoxifen, were significantly reduced in the treatment group. Headaches were less frequently given as a reason for non-compliance by those in the treated group (as compared with control), whereas nausea was cited slightly more often, but neither of these was significant. Mood changes were reported at a similar frequency in the two groups (3%) but were more often a reason for non-compliance in the tamoxifen arm (12 versus 6 cases). Weight gain, another side-effect often attributed to tamoxifen in uncontrolled studies, was also reported significantly less often in the tamoxifen group (7% versus 11%). The overall changes in measured body weight were not significantly different in the two groups, and body weight change was given as the reason for non-compliance in similar numbers of women (9 versus 6 cases). Overall compliance in this trial has been excellent, and 5-year compliance is projected (by the Kaplan–Meier method) to exceed 75% in the treated arm.

Endometrial cancer

Several trials and studies have reported an excess of endometrial cancer in tamoxifen-treated patients, and the published data from randomized trials are summarized in Table 3. The spread of reported risks is large, ranging from no increase to a sevenfold increase. The Swedish investigators were the first to report an increased risk and the most recent figures from their trial (which used a dose of 40 mg/day for 2 or 5 years) are 19 cases in the tamoxifen arm versus 3 in the control arm (29). More recently, the NSABP B-14 (placebo-controlled) trial of 5 years of tamoxifen at the more conventional dose of 20 mg/day reported 15 cases in the treated arm versus 2 in the control group. The most striking feature of these data is the low number of cases in the control group, since about seven would have been expected based on national rates. If allowance

is made for this, these results are compatible with a two- to threefold risk for 5 years of treatment, which is what is suggested from the results in other trials as a whole. A large Dutch case–control study (30) has also reached similar conclusions. In this study a relative risk of 2.4 was found for more than 2 years of use and the projected risk for 5 years or more was threefold. There have been some deaths from endometrial cancer, but most cases have been found at an early stage and are of low malignancy grade, suggesting that the prognosis is similar to or better than the average for endometrial cancer, and is certainly better than that for breast cancer. A few high-grade endometrial carcinomas and sarcomas have been reported (31), but these appear to be very rare

Table 3. Incidence of endometrial cancer in post-menopausal patients in published randomized, controlled studies

Study (Ref.)	Dose (mg/day)	Treatment duration in years (follow-up)	Tamoxifen Cases/no. of patients	Tamoxifen Frequency (%)	Controls Cases/no. of patients	Controls Frequency (%)
NSABP B-14 (52)	20	5 (7)	15/1419	1.06	2/1424	0.14
NATO (70)[a]	20	2 (8)	0/481	0	0/495	0
Scottish (71, 72)	20	5 (10)	1/476	0.21	2/470	0.43
Christie (73)	20	1 (13)	1/282	0.4	1/306	0.3
ECOG [a]	20	2 (5)	1/91	1.1	1/90	1.1
Southwest Oncology Group (74)	20		4/641	0.6	0/325	0
Total	**20**		**22/3390**	**0.65**	**6/3110**	**0.19**
Toronto-Edmonton	30	2 (5.8)	0/198		1/202	0.5
Danish study (69, 75)	30	48 weeks (8 years)	7/864	0.8	2/846	0.2
Copenhagen (76)	30	2 (9)	2/52	3.85	0/52	0
Total	**30**		**9/1114**	**0.81**	**3/1100**	**0.27**
Swedish study (29)	40	2 or 5 (7)	19/931	2.0	3/915	0.33
Overall total	**20–40**		**50/5435**	**0.92***	**12/5125**	**0.23**

Comparison with control groups: *P < 0.0001.
[a] Data quoted by Nayfield et al. (9) from information provided by Zeneca Pharmaceuticals.

Table 4. Summary of three studies of endometrial changes in post-menopausal breast cancer patients treated with or without tamoxifen (32, 33, 34)

	Finland		United Kingdom		Israel	
	Tamoxifen	**Control**	**Tamoxifen**	**Control**	**Tamoxifen**	**Control**
Total studied	51	52	61	50	93	20
Endometrial thickness ≥ 5 mm	43 (84%)	10 (19%)	28 (46%)	6 (12%)	88 (95%)	8 (40%)
Polyps present	17 (36%)	5 (10%)	5 (8%)	1 (2%)	5 (5%)	
Histopathology						
Atrophic	31 (69%)	41 (79%)	37 (61%)	45 (90%)	60 (65%)	16 (80%)
Proliferative	11 (25%)	4 (8%)	14 (23%)	5 (10%)	23 (25%)	4 (20%)
Hyperplastic	2 (4%)	0 (0%)	10 (16%)	0 (0%)	2 (2%)	0 (0%)
Cancer	1 (2%)	2 (4%)	0 (0%)	0 (0%)	3 (3%)	0 (0%)
Insufficient sample	6 (12%)	5 (10%)	–	–	–	–

and it is not possible to assess their importance or their relation to tamoxifen at this stage.

Several studies have reported abnormal uterine pathology in post-menopausal women receiving tamoxifen. In many cases, these reports are based on referred symptomatic patients, so it is not possible to assess the prevalence of these conditions. Lahti et al. (32), Kedar et al. (33) and Cohen et al. (34) have examined unselected post-menopausal breast cancer patients, of whom about one-half were treated with tamoxifen (except for Cohen et al. whose study had much fewer controls). In these studies, a proliferative endometrium was much more common in tamoxifen-treated women, consistent with its oestrogen agonist properties (Table 4). Polyps and atypical hyperplasia were also significantly more common in the tamoxifen groups.

Almost all of the cases of endometrial cancer have been in post-menopausal women, despite a reasonable proportion of pre-menopausal women in some of the studies (e.g. NSABP B-14, NATO, CRCII). This is in keeping with the oestrogen agonist properties of tamoxifen and suggests that any special monitoring or prophylaxis need only be considered for post-menopausal women. Women in prevention trials will be younger and more likely to be pre-menopausal than those with breast cancer in the adjuvant studies, which limits the size of this problem in a preventive setting. The

appropriate screening protocols for post-menopausal women are still uncertain (35, 36) and the value of trans-vaginal ultrasound and/or endometrial biopsy is still under investigation. However, all are agreed that prompt investigation of any vaginal bleeding or discharge in post-menopausal women is essential.

Liver cancer

Several studies have shown that tamoxifen initiates liver adenomas and carcinomas in some species of rats (37, 38, 39) but not in others (40) where it was found to have only promotional activity. DNA adducts, presumably to tamoxifen metabolites, have also been reported (41, 42). These studies have used doses well in excess of the standard dose given to women and are difficult to extrapolate to the human situation. For example, in the lowest dose (5 mg/kg) of the study by Greaves et al. (37), overall survival was significantly better in tamoxifen-treated rats, due to reduction in breast cancers, pituitary cancers and chronic renal disease. One study has looked for DNA adducts in liver biopsies of women taking tamoxifen, and no increase over background levels could be detected (43).

Tamoxifen has been found to inhibit this promotional effect of oestradiol in rats (44), and one trial has reported a beneficial effect of tamoxifen in the treatment of human liver tumours (45).

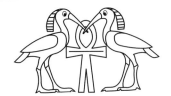

International Breast Cancer Intervention Study

Eligibility Criteria for Entry

Age 45–65, with one or more of the following:

1. Breast cancer in mother, sister or daughter diagnosed at the age of 50 or younger.
2. Mother, sister or daughter who developed cancer in both breasts.
3. Two or more close blood relatives (mother, sisters, daughters, aunts or grandmothers) who have had breast cancer at any age.
4. Having no children and a mother or sister who developed breast cancer.
5. Having had a benign biopsy with proliferative disease and a mother, sister or daughter who developed breast cancer.
6. Lobular carcinoma in situ.
7. Atypical ductal or lobular hyperplasia diagnosed at biopsy.

Age 40–44, with one or more of the following:

1. Two or more close blood relatives (mother, sisters, daughters, aunts or grandmothers) who developed breast cancer at age 50 or younger.
2. Mother, sister or daughter who developed cancer in both breasts, with first cancer diagnosed at age of 50 or younger.
3. Having no children and a mother or sister who developed breast cancer at age 40 or younger.
4. Having had a benign biopsy with proliferative disease and a mother, sister or daughter who developed breast cancer at age 40 or younger.
5. Lobular carcinoma in situ.
6. Atypical ductal or lobular hyperplasia diagnosed at biopsy.

Age 35–39, with one or more of the following:

1. Two or more first degree blood relatives (mother, sisters or daughters) who developed breast cancer at age 50 or less.
2. Mother or sister who developed breast cancer in both breasts, with first cancer diagnosed at age 40 or younger.
3. Lobular carcinoma in situ.

Exclusions

1. Pregnant or at pregnancy risk. Pre or peri-menopausal women must use non-hormonal contraceptive during tamoxifen therapy.
2. A previous cancer, except in situ cervix or basal cell carcinoma of skin.
3. Life expectancy of less than 10 years, or other medical condition more serious than the risk of breast cancer.
4. Psychologically or physically unsuitable for five years tamoxifen/placebo therapy.
5. Current treatment with anti-coagulants.
6. A previous deep vein thrombosis or pulmonary embolus.
7. Current tamoxifen use.

Fig. 4. Criteria for participation or exclusion in the International Breast Cancer Intervention Study.

The available epidemiological evidence is also reassuring as far as it goes. Only nine cases of primary liver cancer (or bile duct cancer) have been reported in trials (46, 68, 69). Three of these were in control patients who did not receive tamoxifen, compared with four cases in direct comparison arms. The other two occurred in tamoxifen-treated patients who did not have direct controls. The intense interest in this question since 1987 has led to only one reported case (47), and even in this case, chemotherapy was also given. A large study (48) from nine population-based cancer registries in the United States has also failed to detect any increase in liver tumours in women with breast cancer after the introduction of tamoxifen in 1977. However, there is a limited amount of long-term follow-up, so there is still uncertainty about the long-term risks. There are also two reports of liver damage (49, 50), but this seems to be extremely rare in view of the considerable exposure to this drug.

Other cancers

Second tumours are notoriously under-reported and the adjuvant trials were not designed to record them. The potential for biased reporting based on exposure to any drug (which is the basis of most adverse event reporting schemes) limits the usefulness of studies of other cancers following breast cancer unless a placebo control is used. Excesses and deficits of different cancers have been reported in different trials, but an overview found a similar number of cancers in treated and control arms (51). No significant differences have been observed in the one reported placebo-controlled trial (52).

Thromboembolic events

Early studies and case reports suggested an excess of thromboembolic events in patients treated with tamoxifen, but in almost all cases either prednisone or cytotoxic chemotherapy was also given. In a placebo-controlled study of tamoxifen alone, Fisher et al. (53) found an excess of phlebitis in the tamoxifen arm (12 versus 2 events) and there was one fatal pulmonary embolism. In contrast, in a Swedish study, Rutqvist & Mattson (14) found little difference in the rates of these events (49 for the tamoxifen arm versus 45 for the control). Several studies have found small reductions in antithrombin III levels, especially in post-menopausal women, but they have rarely dropped below the normal range

and Powles et al. (28) did not observe a significant effect on the fibrinogen/antithrombin III ratio.

Ocular toxicity

A characteristic 'tamoxifen retinopathy' has been reported in which opaque white filaments are formed in the retina, leading to macular oedema and loss of visual acuity. Many of the reported cases were at relatively high doses (40–240 mg daily), and even at these doses this phenomenon has been very rare. However, a few cases have been reported at 20 mg. In most cases, the vision has reverted to normal after cessation of treatment. It has also been suggested that tamoxifen might cause cataracts (54), but the one controlled study found no evidence for this (55). One prospective study has reported reversible decreased visual acuity (56), but two subsequent reports have not confirmed this (57, 58). Serious visual disturbances are extremely rare.

Other toxicity

Ovarian cysts appear to be increased in premenopausal women (28, 34), but they are asymptomatic and are only detected by ultrasound screening. Their clinical importance is unclear since there is no evidence of an increase in ovarian cancer thus far. A case of fatal neutropenia has also been reported (59), but again this appears to be extremely rare.

Table 5. Projected effects over 10 years of giving tamoxifen for 5 years to 10 000 women aged 50 with 2.5-fold relative risk of breast cancer	
	No. of women
Benefits	
Breast cancer (incidence down 40%)	200 (↓)
Ischaemic heart disease (down 20%)	
Incidence	90 (↓)
Mortality	30 (↓)
Spinal fractures (down 33%)	50 (↓)
Risks	
Endometrial cancer (up threefold)	50 (↑)
Thromboembolic disease (blood clots)	20 (↑)
Serious eye problems (retinopathy)	1 (↑)
Liver cancer (liver damage)	< 1 (↑) (?)

Table 6. Age distributions for women at time of entry into tamoxifen prevention trial

Age (years)	Middle age cohort	Younger age cohort
35–39	5%	5%
40–44	5%	10%
45–49	30%	40%
50–54	25%	30%
55–59	20%	10%
60–64	15%	5%

Trial design

Need for trials

The fact that breast cancer is the most common cancer in women and is still increasing rapidly on a worldwide scale strongly favours new initiatives in this area. Modest gains in survival have been made by using tamoxifen and cytotoxic agents, and mammographic screening appears to reduce mortality by about 30% in post-menopausal women. However, screening appears to be much less effective at younger ages. Neither treatment nor screening has any effect on the incidence of disease, nor do they have a large impact on breast cancer mortality in public health terms. The possibilities for prevention with tamoxifen have been widely recognized and three trials are now in progress – one in the United States and Canada (60), one in Italy (61) for hysterectomized women (due to concerns about endometrial cancer), and an international trial coordinated from the United Kingdom. All trials are offering tamoxifen or placebo for 5 years. It is generally agreed that the first trials should be conducted in women who are at increased risk of breast cancer, and in practical terms this usually results in recruiting women with a family history of breast cancer or a previous benign lesion that indicates an increased risk of cancer. The entry criteria for the United Kingdom-based trial are shown in Fig. 4. In broad terms they offer participation to women aged 45–65 years with at least a twofold relative risk, women aged 40–44 years with at least a fourfold risk and women aged 35–39 years with a very high risk (approximately 10-fold). Using this risk profile, about 15 000 participants are needed to detect reliably a one-third reduction in incidence within 10 years, and about 50 000 women are needed to see a similar reduction in mortality. Similar but more detailed criteria are used in the American trial (60). For this trial, women aged 60 years or more are eligible without any risk factors and younger women are eligible if they have risk factors that increase their risk to at least that of a normal 60-year-old woman using a multivariate model developed by Gail et al. (62). Entry into the Italian trial is restricted to hysterectomized women aged 50–60 years, but no risk factors are required (61). Thus, it is clear that all three trials will need to be combined to examine the mortality question with appropriate power.

Pre-menopausal versus post-menopausal women

There has been discussion (15) about whether it is appropriate to include pre-menopausal women in prevention trials. As a baseline, the projected 10-year risks and benefits for 10 000 women aged 50 years with a 2.5-fold increased risk are shown in Table 5. It is emphasized that these are projections based on currently available evidence and a trial is essential to confirm their validity. Breast cancer emerges as the most common event and, based on

Table 7. Projected major end-points in 10 years for 10 000 women treated in a chemoprevention trial versus 10 000 controls, for two age distributions

	Tamoxifen (No.)	Control (No.)	Difference (No.)
Breast cancer incidence			
(down 40%)			
Older	300	500	200 (↓)
Younger	283	471	188 (↓)
Endometrial cancer incidence			
(up threefold over age 50)			
Older	91	31	60 (↑)
Younger	78	28	50 (↑)
Myocardial infarction incidence			
(down 20% over age 50)			
Older	316	389	73 (↓)
Younger	229	279	50 (↓)

a 40% reduction in breast cancer, a tripling of endometrial cancer and United Kingdom incidence rates, the reduction in incidence of breast cancer is four times greater than the increase in endometrial cancer. Furthermore, since the prognosis for breast cancer is much worse than for endometrial cancer, the ratio in terms of mortality is even better, and is probably around 10 : 1. In addition, any increase in endometrial cancer is more than compensated for by the larger reduction in the incidence of myocardial infarction, where again the ratio is more favourable if mortality is considered. The reduction in spinal fractures is based on extrapolation from results of HRT usage, where larger benefits are seen but larger effects on bone density also occur (63). We have considered only spinal fractures, although hip fractures may also be reduced (23). The effects on bone density are more likely to influence fractures occurring more than 10 years after entry as this is a very age-dependent factor. Assuming a one-third decrease, the lifetime reduction is estimated to be 10 times larger (i.e. a reduction of 500 spinal fractures in 10000 treated women). The remaining risks related to thromboembolic disease, eye problems, liver cancer and liver disease are poorly quantified and the corresponding estimates are crude, but they can be seen to be much less important than the factors already considered.

For pre-menopausal women, the minimum rates of breast cancer in the control groups will be larger than for post-menopausal women, because of the higher relative risk required for eligibility. Although there is much less evidence available on this question, the reduction in recurrence rates and mortality in pre-menopausal women was similar to that for post-menopausal women in the worldwide overview (7; Table 3), and a recent publication supports the value of giving tamoxifen for 2 years in addition to chemotherapy in pre-menopausal women (64). Also in the NSABP B-14 trial, there was a greater reduction in new contralateral tumours in premenopausal women than in post-menopausal women. Thus the available evidence suggests that the absolute reduction in breast cancer incidence may be even greater for eligible pre-menopausal women in the trial. However, they will probably not benefit in terms of bone density, and any reduction in cardiovascular disease is more speculative and likely to be smaller. The problems with endometrial cancer do not appear to affect pre-menopausal

women, but any problems with ovarian cysts will be concentrated within this group. It is unclear whether thromboembolic problems will differentially affect this group. Overall, the benefit : risk ratio for this group depends critically upon the effects on breast cancer incidence, as the benefits in terms of ischaemic heart disease and fractures will be minimal. The uncertainties about the effect of tamoxifen on the fetus are also a concern for younger premenopausal women.

In summary, the projected 10-year effects on breast cancer, endometrial cancer and heart disease of 20 mg tamoxifen given to 10 000 women for 5 years, following an 'older' or 'younger' age distribution (which is believed to bracket the true age distribution for the United Kingdom prevention trial; Table 6), are shown in Table 7.

Tamoxifen analogues

Several analogues of tamoxifen have been synthesized and evaluated, including toremifene, droloxifene, and pyrrolidino-tamoxifen. Of these, toremifene has been the most fully studied and it has been shown not to produce DNA adducts in rat liver or to cause liver cancers in rats (65). However, it appears to have the same oestrogen agonist properties as tamoxifen and thus is likely to produce the same side-effects in the endometrium. In view of the increasing evidence that liver tumours are not a cause for concern in humans, the currently available analogues do not appear to have much to offer, and until much more experience is gathered in the adjuvant setting, their use in a preventive trial setting is not appropriate.

Genetic testing

Genetic testing offers the possibility to determine more accurately the risk of breast cancer in an individual woman. In some cases, such as for BRCA1 gene carriers in breast cancer families, the lifetime risk is so high (70%) that more extreme measures than tamoxifen prophylaxis (e.g. bilateral mastectomy) may be appropriate. However, mutations of this gene in the general population are likely to confer a substantially lower risk, and it is likely that the majority of familial aggregation is due to other lower risk genes (e.g. AT-heterozygotes) where bilateral mastectomy is considered too extreme and less drastic approaches are called for. Thus, overall, genetic testing is likely to increase the number of women who are known to be at sufficient risk to justify chemoprevention.

Conclusion

Prevention appears to offer the best hope of making a substantial impact on the morbidity and mortality due to breast cancer. On a worldwide scale, this problem will only become larger in the next few decades. At the moment tamoxifen is the only agent sufficiently well explored to justify large-scale trials, and three trials are in progress worldwide. However, this is only the first step in developing preventive strategies. Their success will stimulate development of similar but more specific agents for prevention, in addition to providing further incentives for funding research into genetic and other risk factors for this disease, and for developing additional strategies, possibly based on dietary intervention (66, 67) or new oral contraceptives which reduce the risk of breast cancer.

References

1 Parkin DM, Pisani P, Ferlay J. Estimates of the worldwide incidence of eighteen major cancers in 1985. *Int J Cancer*, 1993, 54:594–606.

2 Pisani P, Parkin DM, Ferlay J. Estimates of the worldwide mortality from eighteen major cancers in 1985. Implications for prevention and projections of future burden. *Int J Cancer*, 1993, 55:891–903.

3 De Ridder CM et al. Dietary habits, sexual maturation, and plasma hormones in pubertal girls: a longitudinal study. *Am J Clin Nutr*, 1991, 54:805–813.

4 Spicer DV et al. Changes in mammographic densities induced by hormonal contraceptive designed to reduce breast cancer risk. *J Natl Cancer Inst*, 1994, 86:431–436.

5 Trichopoulos D et al. Menopause and breast cancer risk. *J Natl Cancer Inst*, 1972, 48:1347–1360.

6 Furr B, Jordan V. The pharmacology and clinical uses of tamoxifen. *Pharmac Ther*, 1984, 25:127–205.

7 Early Breast Cancer Trialists' Collaborative Group. Systemic treatment of early breast cancer by hormonal, cytotoxic, or immune therapy. *Lancet*, 1992, 339:1–15.

8 Cuzick J, Baum M. Tamoxifen and contralateral breast cancer. *Lancet*, 1985, ii:282.

9 Nayfield SG et al. Potential role of tamoxifen in the prevention of breast cancer. *J Natl Cancer Inst*, 1991, 83:1450–1459.

10 Baum M, Houghton J, Riley D. Results of the cancer research campaign adjuvant trial for perioperative cyclophosphamide and long-term tamoxifen in early breast cancer reported at the tenth year of follow-up. *Acta Oncol*, 1992, 31:251–257.

11 Jordan VC. *Chemosuppression of breast cancer with tamoxifen: Laboratory evidence and future clinical investigation*. Madison, WI, University of Wisconsin Press, 1988.

12 Wiseman H. *Tamoxifen: Molecular Basis of Use in Cancer Treatment and Prevention*. Chichester, Wiley, 1994.

13 McDonald CC, Stewart HJ for the Scottish Breast Cancer Committee. Fatal myocardial infarction in the Scottish adjuvant tamoxifen trial. *Br Med J*, 1991, 303: 435–437.

14 Rutqvist LE, Mattson A. Cardiac and thromboembolic morbidity among postmenopausal women with early-stage breast cancer in a randomised trial of adjuvant tamoxifen. *J Natl Cancer Inst*, 1993, 85:1398–1406.

15 Love RR, Mamby CC, Feyzi JM. Tamoxifen-induced decreases in total cholesterol with 2 weeks of treatment. *J Natl Cancer Inst*, 1993, 85:1344–1345.

16 Cuzick J et al. Long term effects of tamoxifen. *Eur J Cancer*, 1993, 29A:15–21.

17 Wiseman H et al. Tamoxifen inhibits lipid peroxidation in cardiac microsomes. *Biochem Pharm*, 1993, 45:1851–1855.

18 Wiseman H et al. Protective actions of tamoxifen and 4-hydroxytamoxifen against oxidative damage to human low-density lipoproteins: a mechanism accounting for the cardioprotective action of tamoxifen? *Biochem J*, 1993, 292:635–638.

19 Thangaraju M et al. Effects of tamoxifen on plasma lipids and lipoproteins in postmenopausal women with breast cancer. *Cancer*, 1994, 73:659–663.

20 Love RR et al. Effects of tamoxifen on bone mineral density in post menopausal women with breast cancer. *New Engl J Med*, 1992, 326:852–856.

21 Turken S et al. Effects of tamoxifen on spinal bone density in women with breast cancer. *J Natl Cancer Inst*, 1989, 81:1086–1088.

22 Ryan WG, Wolter J, Bagdade JD. Apparent beneficial effects of tamoxifen on bone mineral content in patients with breast cancer: preliminary study. *Osteoporosis Int*, 1991, 2:39–41.

23 Ward RL et al. Tamoxifen reduces bone turnover and prevents lumber spine and proximal femoral bone loss in early postmenopausal women. *Bone & Mineral*, 1993, 22:87–94.

24 Kristensen B et al. Tamoxifen and bone metabolism in postmenopausal low-risk breast cancer patients: A randomized study. *J Clin Oncol*, 1994, 12:992–997.

25 Gotfredson A, Christiansen C, Palshof T. The effect of tamoxifen on bone mineral content in premenopausal women with breast cancer. *Cancer*, 1984, 53:853–857.

26 Fentiman I et al. Bone mineral content of women receiving tamoxifen for mastalgia. *Br J Cancer*, 1989, 60:262–264.

27 O'Brien M, Powles TJ. Tamoxifen in the prevention of breast cancer. Are the risks likely to outweigh the benefits? *Drug Saf*, 1994, 10:1–4.

28 Powles TJ et al. The Royal Marsden Hospital pilot tamoxifen chemoprevention trial. *Breast Cancer Res Treat*, 1994, 31:73–83.

29 Fornander T et al. Oestrogenic effects of adjuvant tamoxifen in postmenopausal breast cancer. *Eur J Cancer*, 1993, 29A:497–500.

30 van Leeuwen FE, Benraadt J, Coebergh JWW et al. Risk of endometrial cancer after tamoxifen treatment of breast cancer. *Lancet*, 1994, 343:448–452.

31 Magriples U et al. High-grade endometrial carcinoma in tamoxifen-treated breast cancer patients. *J Clin Oncol*, 1993, 11:485–490.

32 Lahti E et al. Endometrial changes in postmenopausal breast cancer patients receiving tamoxifen. *Obstet Gynecol*, 1993, 81:660–664.

33 Kedar RP et al. Effects of tamoxifen on uterus and ovaries of premenopausal women in a randomised breast cancer prevention trial. *Lancet*, 1994, 343:1318–1321.

34 Cohen I et al. Endometrial changes with tamoxifen: Comparison between tamoxifen-treated and nontreated asymptomatic, postmenopausal breast cancer patients. *Gynecol Oncol*, 1994, 52:185–190.

35 Bissett D, Davis JA, George WD. Gynaecological monitoring during tamoxifen therapy. *Lancet*, 1994, 344:1244.

36 Neven P et al. Tamoxifen and the uterus. *Br Med J*, 1994, 309:1313–1314.

37 Greaves P et al. Ten year carcinogenicity study of tamoxifen in Alderley park wistar-derived rats. *Cancer Res*, 1993, 53:3919–3924.

38 Hirsimaki P et al. Tamoxifen induces hepatocellular carcinoma in rat liver: a 1-year study with two antioestrogens. *Arch Toxicol*, 1993, 67:49–54.

39 Williams GM et al. The triphenyl-ethylene drug tamoxifen is a strong liver carcinogen in the rat. *Carcinogenesis*, 1993, 14:315–317.

40 Dragan YP et al. Studies of tamoxifen as a promoter of hepatocarcinogenesis in Fischer 344 rats. *Breast Cancer Res Treat*, 1994, 13:11–25.

41 Han X, Liehr J. Induction of covalent DNA adducts in rodents by tamoxifen. *Cancer Res*, 1992, 52:1360–1363.

42 White INH et al. Genotoxic potential of tamoxifen and analogues in female fischer F344/n rats, DBA/2 and C57BL/6 mice and in human MCL-5 cells. *Carcinogenesis*, 1992, 13:2197–2203.

43 Martin EA et al. A comparison of p-postlabelled tamoxifen liver DNA adducts in rats, mice and breast cancer patients. *Toxicologist*, 1994, 14: A1602.

44 Yager JD, Shi YE. Synthetic estrogens and tamoxifen as promoters of hepatocarcinogenesis. *Prev Med*, 1991, 20:27–37.

45 Farinati F et al. Prospective controlled trial with antiestrogen drug tamoxifen in patients with unresectable hepatocellular carcinoma. *Dig Dis Sci*, 1992, 37:659–662.

46 Rutqvist LE, Johansson H, Signomklao T et al. Adjuvant tamoxifen therapy for early stage breast cancer and second primary malignancies. *J Natl Cancer Inst*, 1995, 87:645–651.

47 Johnstone AJ, Sarkar TK, Hussey JK. Primary hepatocellular carcinoma in a patient with breast carcinoma. *Clin Oncol*, 1991, 3:180–181.

48 Muhlemann K, Cook LS, Weiss NS. The incidence of hepatocellular carcinoma in US white women with breast cancer after the introduction of tamoxifen in 1977. *Breast Cancer Res Treat*, 1994, 30:201–204.

49 Blackburn A et al. Tamoxifen and liver damage. *Br Med J*, 1984, 289:288.

50 Ching CK, Smith PG, Long RG. Tamoxifen-associated hepatocellular damage and agranulocytosis. *Lancet*, 1992, 339:940.

51 Jackson IM, Litherland S, Wakeling AE. Tamoxifen and other antiestrogens. In: Powles TJ, Smith IE, eds. *Medical Management of Breast Cancer*. London, Martin Dunizt, 1991.

52 Fisher B et al. Endometrial cancer in tamoxifen-treated breast cancer patients: Findings from the National Surgical Adjuvant Breast and Bowel Project (NSABP) B-14. *J Natl Cancer Inst*, 1994, 86:527–537.

53 Fisher B et al. A randomised clinical trial evaluating tamoxifen in the treatment of patients with node-negative breast cancer who have estrogen-receptor-positive tumours. *N Engl J Med*, 1989, 320:479–484.

54 Zhang JJ et al. Tamoxifen blocks chloride channels: A possible mechanism for cataract formation. *J Clin Inv*, 1994, 94:1690–1697.

55 Longstaff S et al. A controlled study of the ocular effects of tamoxifen in conventional dosage in the treatment of breast carcinoma. *Eur J Cancer Clin Oncol*, 1989, 25:1805–1808.

56 Pavlidis N et al. Clear evidence that long-term, low-dose tamoxifen treatment can induce ocular toxicity. *Cancer*, 1992, 69:2961–2964.

57 Heier JS et al. Screening for ocular toxicity in asymptomatic patients treated with tamoxifen. *Am J Ophth*, 1994, 17:772–775.

58 Locher D et al. Retinal changes associated with tamoxifen treatment for breast cancer. *Inv Ophth & Vis Sci*, 1994, 35:1526.

59 Mike V, Currie VE, Gee TS. Fatal neutropenia associated with long-term tamoxifen therapy. *Lancet*, 1994, 344:541–542.

60 Redmond CK, Costantino JP. Design and current status of the NSABP breast cancer prevention trial (BCPT). In: *Proceedings of Adjuvant Therapy of Cancer: Recent Results in Cancer Research*. Berlin, Springer-Verlag Press, 1996.

61 Veronesi U et al. Breast cancer chemoprevention with tamoxifen. A proposed study of the Italian group for cancer prevention. In: De Palo G, Sporn M, Veronesi U, eds. *Progress and Perspectives in Chemoprevention of Cancer*, Vol. 79. New York, Raven Press, 1992.

62 Gail MH et al. Projecting individualized probabilities of developing breast cancer for white females who are being examined annually. *J Natl Cancer Inst*, 1989, 81:1879–1885.

63 Whitehead M, Godfrey V. *Hormone Replacement Therapy*. Edinburgh, Churchill Livingstone, 1992.

64 Cummings FJ et al. Adjuvant tamoxifen versus placebo in elderly women with node-positive breast cancer: Long-term follow-up and causes of death. *J Clin Oncol*, 1993, 11:29–35.

65 Hard GC et al. Major difference in the hepatocarcinogenicity and DNA adduct forming ability between toremifene and tamoxifen in female Crl:CD(BR) rats. *Cancer Res*, 1993, 53:4534–4541.

66 Prentice R L et al. Aspects of the rationale for the women's health trial. *J Natl Cancer Inst*, 1988, 80:802–814.

67 Boyd NF et al. Dietary fat and breast cancer risk: The feasibility of a clinical trial of breast cancer prevention. *Lipids*, 1992, 27:821–826.

68 Ryden S, Ferno M, Moller T et al. Long-term effects of adjuvant tamoxifen and/or radiotherapy. *Acta Oncol*, 1992, 31:271–274.

69 Andersson M, Storm HH, Mouridsen HT. (1991). Incidence of new primary cancers after adjuvant tamoxifen therapy and radiotherapy for early breast cancer. *J Natl Cancer Inst*, 83:1013–1017.

70 NATO (Novaldex Adjuvant Trial Organization). Controlled trial of tamoxifen as a single adjuvant agent in the management of early breast cancer. *Br J Cancer*, 1988, 57:608–611.

71 Stewart HJ, Knight GM. Tamoxifen and the uterus and endometrium. *Lancet*, 1989, i:375–376.

72 Stewart H. The Scottish trial of adjuvant tamoxifen in node-negative breast cancer. *J Natl Cancer Inst Monogr*, 1992, 11:117–120.

73 Ribeiro G, Swindell R. The Christie Hospital Adjuvant Tamoxifen Trial. *J Natl Cancer Inst Monogr*, 1992, 11:121–125.

74 Sunderland MC, Osborne CK. Tamoxifen in premenopausal patients with metastatic breast cancer: a review. *J Clin Oncol*, 1991, 9:1283–1297.

75 Andersson M, Storm HS, Mouridsen HT et al. Carcinogenic effects of adjuvant tamoxifen treatment and radiotherapy for early breast cancer. *Acta Oncol*, 1992, 31:259–263.

76 Palshof T. Adjuvant endocrine therapy in premenopausal and postmenopausal women with breast cancer. Report of the Copenhagen Breast Cancer Trials 1975–1987. Copenhagen, Medi-book, 1988.

77 Rossner S, Walgren A. Serum lipoproteins and proteins after breast cancer surgery and effects of tamoxifen. *Artherosclerosis*, 1984, 52:339–348.

78 Caleffi M, Fentiman I, Clark G et al. Effect of tamoxifen on oestrogen binding, lipid and lipoprotein concentrations and blood clotting parameters in premenopausal women with breast pain. *J Endocrinol*, 1988, 119:335–339.

79 Bruning P, Bonfrer J, Hart A, et al. Tamoxifen, serum lipoproteins and cardiovascular risk. *Br J Cancer*, 1988, 58:497–499.

80 Love RR, Newcomb P, Wiebe D et al. Effects of tamoxifen therapy on lipid and lipoprotein levels in postmenopausal patients with node-negative breast cancer. *J Natl Cancer Inst*, 1990, 82:1327–1332.

81 Dewar JA, Horobin JM, Preece PE et al. Long term effects of tamoxifen on blood lipid values in breast cancer. *Br Med J*, 1992, 305:225–226.

82 Thangaraju M, Ilanchezhian S, Ezhilarasi R et al. Lipid peroxidation and antioxidative enzyme levels in tamoxifen-treated women with breast cancer, in relation to the menopausal status of the patients. *Med Sci Res*, 1993, 21:721–723.

83 Dziewulska-Bokiniec A, Wojtacki J, Skokowski J et al. The effect of tamoxifen on serum cholesterol fractions in breast cancer women. *Neoplasm*, 1994, 41:13–16.

J. Cuzick
Imperial Cancer Research Fund, 61 Lincoln's Inn Fields, London WC2A 3PX, United Kingdom

Chemoprevention of skin cancer

A. Green

Skin cancer is much more common than any other cancer among European populations, yet few data are available regarding the potential effectiveness of chemoprevention of skin tumours. The most promising preventive agents are high-protection sunscreens, but to date their long-term effectiveness has barely been researched in humans, and so there is no firm basis for advocating their use to prevent skin cancer. Antioxidant vitamins have not yet been shown to be effective, but these agents have not been fully investigated, and findings from ongoing trials may clarify their usefulness in skin cancer control. Retinoids may be of benefit to a small number of patients for whom there is a very high risk of skin cancer and who are prepared to tolerate the toxic side-effects that frequently occur with effective doses. Thus the effectiveness of chemopreventive measures against skin cancer, as a complement to photoprotective measures, remains to be established.

Introduction

Surprisingly little research has been undertaken to evaluate the prevention of skin cancer, despite its being by far the most common of all cancers among white populations of European descent. For example, in the Australian population, which has the highest reported occurrence rates, the minimum incidence of the non-melanocytic skin cancers, basal cell carcinoma (BCC) and squamous cell carcinoma (SCC), is estimated to be 977 per 100 000 persons per year (1). This is more than 10 times the combined rates of incidence of the three other major types of cancer – lung, breast and colon cancer. Even in white populations at intermediate risk, such as in the United States, non-melanocytic skin cancers impose an enormous public health burden, with around a million new cases per year (2), while in low-risk white populations the incidence of skin cancer is on the increase. In Switzerland (3), for example, it was around 50 per 100 000 per persons per year in 1984–1985 and appeared to be rising. Cutaneous melanoma is the least common of the major skin cancers, with average incidence rates in Europe of less than

10 per 100 000 persons per year, which is less than one-half the average incidence in Australia. Melanoma causes concern because incidence rates are increasing worldwide, it is often fatal and it commonly affects young people. Indeed, melanomas are among the most malignant of human neoplasms (4).

There are several reasons for the paucity of research into the prevention (including the chemoprevention) of skin cancer compared with the amount of research into much less common cancers such as cancers of the lung or colon. First, non-melanocytic skin cancer has a low case-fatality rate, and is often perceived not to be serious enough to warrant great attention. Secondly, there is sufficient evidence that solar ultraviolet (UV) radiation causes cancer of the skin (5), and since this is the major cause, avoidance of excessive sun exposure has naturally been the mainstay of prevention of skin cancer. The theoretical appeal and prudence of this preventive strategy contrasts with its lack of practical appeal: there is a cultural reluctance among modern Western populations to limit their sun exposure. Thirdly, the necessary evaluation of photoprotection is extremely difficult. Effective chemoprevention would provide a welcome complementary measure to photoprotection in the prevention of skin cancer.

Histogenesis of skin cancer

A BCC is a slowly growing tumour that is usually undifferentiated histologically and rarely metastasizes, although it causes extensive local destruction if inadequately treated. The exact origin (site and cell) of BCCs is unknown, and there is no satisfactory animal model for the disease. A SCC, arising from the keratinizing cells of the epidermis, can metastasize and is the most common type of tumour found after experimental exposure of animals to UV radiation (5). Solar keratoses (SKs) are relatively common dysplastic epidermal lesions which are generally regarded as precursor lesions for SCC, with reported rates of malignant transformation varying from <1:1000 to 20% (6). Unlike BCCs and SCCs, melanomas are not epithelial in origin; they arise from epidermal melanocytes which originate in the neural crest. While the majority of melanomas appear to evolve *de novo*, a small proportion arise in association with benign melanocytic naevi (moles), most frequently in those with histologic dysplasia. The evidence that solar radiation causes melanoma, while compelling (5), is only circumstantial.

Rationale for chemoprevention of skin carcinogenesis

Steps involved in UV carcinogenesis

Ultraviolet irradiation damages nuclear DNA by direct absorption or via photodynamic oxidative mechanisms (7, 8, 9). DNA photolesions are mainly cyclobutane pyrimidine dimers (comprising thymine and cytosine dimers), but they also include (6-4) photoproducts and single-strand breaks (10, 11). Ultraviolet light induces unique mutations, such as CC →TT base changes, which differ from those induced by any other carcinogen, and this specificity results from the predominance of photolesions involving bonds between adjacent pyrimidines on the the same DNA strand (12).

Defective repair of UV-induced pyrimidine dimers is the next critical step in skin tumour induction, as is illustrated by the greatly increased susceptibility to skin cancer of those with the disorder xeroderma pigmentosum (XP), in whom the defective repair is inherited (10). Oncogenes and tumour-suppressor genes are also likely to be involved in skin carcinogenesis. Activated *ras* oncogenes have been identified in human skin cancers (10), and the presence of UV 'signature mutations' in the p53 tumour-suppressor gene in human BCCs, SCCs and UV-induced murine skin tumours (12, 13, 14) is indeed the strongest existing evidence that UV-induced mutations are causally related to the induction and/or progression of these tumours.

Normally, emergent neoplastic cell clones in the epidermis are removed by apoptosis (controlled cell death) or, if not by apoptosis, by immune mechanisms. The importance of immunoregulatory mechanisms in the control of UV-induced cancers in mice was initially demonstrated by Kripke & Fisher (15). Using transplantation experiments, these tumours were shown to be so highly immunogenic that they were unable to escape destruction by the immune system. However, exposure of the host to UV radiation resulted in

abrogation of this immune response, allowing the tumour to grow. The strongest evidence that alterations in immune surveillance mechanisms play a similar role in the pathogenesis of human skin cancer is that organ transplant recipients undergoing immunosuppressive therapy have a greatly increased incidence of skin cancer, in particular SCC (16). Perhaps the best studied of the postulated photoreceptors for immunosuppression in humans are the antigen-presenting cells of the skin, the Langerhans cells. Exposure of these cells to UV radiation causes profound functional and morphological alterations (17, 18), resulting in reduced presentation of antigens introduced into the epidermis, and thus a postulated inability to present neoplastic cells effectively to T-lymphocytes in order to stimulate an appropriate immune response.

Sunscreens

Chemical sunscreens which act as filters preventing transmission of UV radiation to the epidermis and dermis should, *a priori*, protect against all major skin cancers. The effectiveness of a topical sunscreen is assessed by its effectiveness in preventing acute erythema (sunburn), which is caused by UVB and, to a lesser extent, UVA radiation. The sun protection factor (SPF) of a sunscreen is an experimentally derived number that gives an approximation of the protection it affords to the skin against UVB radiation only (no similar convention exists for UVA; 19). (The SPF value is the ratio of UV radiation required to produce recognizable skin erythema in skin that has been protected with a sunscreen to the dose required to have the same effect in unprotected skin under the same conditions; an SPF of 15 or more indicates a maximum protection sunscreen.) A broad-spectrum sunscreen additionally provides some protection against UVA radiation.

The effectiveness of sunscreens is based on two different mechanisms of action, either the absorption of photons, or the physical reflection and scattering of photons. The most widely used photon-absorbing agents are para-aminobenzoic acid (PABA), PABA esters, benzophenones, dibenzoylmethanes, salicylates and cinnamates. While the salicylates and cinnamates absorb in both the UVA and UVB ranges, the two most commonly used chemicals with broad absorption spectra (UVA and UVB) are the benzophenones and the dibenzoylmethanes (19). Besides the absorption spectra of a compound, other determinants of the photoprotectiveness of sunscreens are the substantivity (resistance to removal by sweating or swimming), and the thickness and evenness of application (the standard thickness for SPF determination is 2 mg/cm²). The other types of sunscreen are based on photon-blocking agents such as zinc oxide, titanium dioxide and calamine. These are opaque and although they provide effective protection against UV radiation, they are less cosmetically acceptable since they are visible and occlusive (20).

In addition to conventional sunscreens, UVB sunscreen preparations that contain 5-methoxy-psoralen (5-MOP) extracted from bergamot oil have been marketed. The action of 5-MOP is to enhance photoprotection by stimulating an increase in formation of melanin (tanning pigmentation) in the skin in the presence of solar UVA, but its use is controversial because of its mutagenicity (21).

There is limited laboratory evidence of the effectiveness of sunscreens in preventing DNA photolesions early in cutaneous carcinogenesis. Dimer formation has been shown to be markedly reduced in sunscreen-treated human skin *in situ* compared with untreated skin (22).

Photochemoprotection against DNA damage by UVB sunscreens containing 5-MOP, as measured by unscheduled DNA synthesis and thymine dimer formation, has also been demonstrated (23, 11, 24).

With regard to tumorigenesis, sunscreens have been shown to protect against, or delay, the development of squamous cell carcinoma in several studies involving hairless mice exposed to UV radiation (25, 26, 27, 28). However, there was a loss of photoprotection against chronic damage as the time between treatment of the animals and irradiation increased (29), and sunscreens have recently been reported to be ineffective in protecting against an immmunological effect of UV radiation which enhanced tumour growth in mice injected with melanoma cells following irradiation (30). Other studies suggest that traditional sunscreens still allow low doses of UV radiation to down-regulate the immune system (7). Indeed, it has been proposed that the increasing and widespread use of sunscreens is causing rather than mitigating the rising incidence rates of skin cancer (31).

Antioxidants

Given the general and multiple carcinogenic properties of oxy-radicals, namely that they can cause permanent structural DNA damage and activate cytoplasmic transduction pathways related to growth, differentiation and cell death, it would seem that antioxidants could potentially act as anticarcinogens at multiple stages, although knowing the role of a single agent in the target tissue will depend on the interplay of the multiple antioxidant tissue components and the particular carcinogen involved (9). There is a vast amount of laboratory-based evidence that antioxidant micronutrients (β-carotene, vitamins A,C and E) prevent or retard carcinogenesis, including photocarcinogenesis (reviewed in 32, 33, 34). The capacities of β-carotene and other carotenoids to destroy free radicals may also partly explain their observed immuno-enhancement properties (7, 35, 36).

Retinoids

Numerous mechanisms for the action of retinoids as anticarcinogens in the skin have been proposed, in particular the promotion of cellular differentiation (37). Retinoids may increase epidermal thickness, and thus decrease UV transmission, via an increase in epidermal growth factor receptors (7), and administration in the promotion stage appears to counteract various cellular changes associated with neoplastic transformation, e.g. decrease in cell surface fibronectin and anchorage-independent growth (37). Furthermore, vitamin A and retinoids can act as potent immunoregulatory agents: in mice, a diet enriched in vitamin A acetate increased their ability to respond effectively to tumour antigens and resist tumour growth (38); and in humans, an increase in Langerhan's cells was observed following a topical treatment (39).

Effectiveness of chemopreventive agents in humans

Topical sunscreens

Sunscreens and solar keratoses. In a randomized controlled trial carried out among 431 subjects over 40 years of age in Australia, the regular application of a high-protection sunscreen to the head, neck, forearms and hands was reported to reduce the mean number of SKs and increase the mean number of lesions which remitted during the course of one Australian summer (40). However, this outcome could have been weighted by a favourable response occurring among the typically small minority who carry the majority of prevalent solar keratoses in the Australian population. Adverse reactions to the sunscreen were reported in 19% of this study population; most of these were irritant reactions and only a few were allergic in nature (no person was allergic to the active ingredients in the sunscreen; *41*). Currently, there is no evidence that sunscreens protect against the development of skin cancer, although an ongoing population-based randomized trial concerning the prevention of skin cancer and its precursors, which is being conducted among some 1600 residents of a Queensland community *inter alia*, addresses this question (*42*). It is hypothesized that primary prevention of skin cancer is possible in adults by reducing UV exposure that promotes skin cancer, despite degenerative and premalignant changes that may already have arisen from past exposure.

Antioxidant vitamins

β-carotene and BCC/SCC. Interpretation of the single retrospective hospital-based study that showed an inverse association between serum β-carotene and skin cancer is problematic (*43*). Several prospective studies of pre-diagnostic dietary intake or plasma levels of β-carotene have been reported, but no significant associations with subsequent skin cancer have been found (*44, 45, 46, 47*). Most of these studies involved only modest numbers of skin cancer cases, and in none of these prospective studies were subjects physically examined for skin cancer, raising the possibility of incomplete reporting of its occurrence.

The only published trial of chemoprevention of skin cancer was a randomized double-blind multicentre trial conducted in the United States in patients who had a history of biopsy-proven BCCs or SCCs (*48, 49*). A total of 1805 patients, 35% of those identified as eligible, entered the trial, which involved taking one capsule daily containing either 50 mg β-carotene or a placebo. Compliance in taking the capsules and interim treatment of skin lesions were monitored by a questionnaire every 4 months; skin examinations by a dermatologist were undertaken annually. Results after 5 years of follow-up showed no difference between treatment groups in the rate of occurrence of the first histologically confirmed skin cancer, either

overall (relative rate of 1.05, 95% confidence interval, 0.91–1.22) or considering only those skin cancers appearing in the fifth year of the trial (relative rate 1.11). Furthermore, the mean numbers of new skin cancers per patient-year were not significantly different between the groups, and treatment did not reduce skin cancer in patients who smoked cigarettes or in those whose baseline serum β-carotene levels were relatively low.

These data, although the strongest available evidence regarding the chemoprevention of skin cancer, cannot be considered conclusive. The subjects were a highly selected patient group, mostly males, all of whom had at least one previous skin cancer. While recurrent primary skin tumours may be a good model for a chemoprevention trial in some regards (the lesion is easily measured and there is a short latent period; *50*), carcinogenesis in this setting may not reflect the natural history of skin cancer in general. That is, the steps involved in cutaneous UV-carcinogenesis, even in the late stages, may be different among those of similar age affected *ab initio*. Indeed, the risk of subsequent skin cancer in the US study population (*49*) was found to be 50% at 5 years. Risk was higher among those who lived in California (compared with Minnesota and New Hampshire) and those who had severe actinic damage (*51*). The results suggest that sun exposure is important in the final stages of skin carcinogenesis as well as the early stages, but no allowance, beyond study centre, was made in the adjusted analyses for possible differences in sun exposure between the treatment groups. In addition, the process of skin carcinogenesis was well advanced and thus the potential for cancer prevention may have been extremely limited in the study group as a whole. Ongoing trials include the Nambour Skin Cancer Prevention Trial (*42*), in which a daily dose of 30 mg β-carotene or a placebo has been randomly allocated to some 1600 residents of Nambour. One outcome measure will be based on the calculated cumulative incidence of skin cancer over a period of 3–5 years, together with the change in prevalence of solar keratoses. Since the study population is a highrisk general population rather than a selected patient population as in previous studies (*49*), this trial should provide a superior test of chemoprevention for use in public health control programmes.

β-carotene and melanoma. There has been little consideration of diet or dietary micronutrients in relation to the risk of melanoma, and only two comprehensive analytic assessments of diet and melanoma are available (*52, 53*). One (*52*) was a case–control study based on patients attending a Boston hospital's pigmented lesion clinic. This study reported inverse relations with dietary antioxidants, β-carotene and vitamin E, but the choice of controls was not optimal since they were patients with suspicious pigmented lesions (the strongest risk determinants of melanoma). The small numbers of subjects in the other case–control study (*53*), and the lack of available data on sun exposure in both, mean that the findings are only preliminary. The value of the serological data from the Boston study, which showed no significant associations with plasma levels of retinol, α-carotene, β-carotene, lycopene or α-tocopherol, are similarly limited. The only study to have reported a significant and inverse association between serum β-carotene and α-tocopherol, and subsequent risk of melanoma was a nested case–control study of 39 268 Finnish men and women participating in a national health survey (*54*). However, the results were based on only 10 cases of melanoma, and thus, once again, no firm conclusions can be drawn. No salient randomized trials have been undertaken, and so there is no good evidence to suggest that chemopreventive agents are effective in reducing the occurrence of melanoma.

Retinoids

Oral isotretinoin and BCC/SCC. Of seven patients with XP who were treated with high doses of isotretinoin (13-cis-retinoic acid: 2 mg/kg daily) and protected from sun exposure, five (aged 10–39 years) who tolerated the protocol showed a significant reduction in new tumours over a 2-year period, with a rebound effect on cessation of therapy (*55*). All the patients experienced typical mucocutaneous toxic effects (cheilitis, marked xerosis of skin), increased conjunctivitis and blepharitis, and showed variably elevated or abnormal serum levels of triglycerides and liver function. Several patients experienced arthralgia of the spine and small joints. Since the high doses were too toxic for long-term therapy, a daily dose of 0.5 mg/kg was administered for 1 year, with variable effectiveness but with less severe toxic effects (*56*). It was concluded

that isotretinoin acts at a late stage in carcinogenesis with rapid onset and loss of effect coincident with therapy (*56*), and that it may be of short-lived benefit, despite the substantial toxicity, in patients with or without XP who are developing numerous new skin cancers each year.

On the basis of case reports in which isotretinoin in high doses appeared to have a prophylactic effect on skin cancer but with high toxicity (*57*), the effectiveness of low doses of isotretinoin in preventing additional BCCs was evaluated in a clinical trial (*58*). At eight centres in the United States, 981 patients, aged 40–75 years and with two or more previously treated BCCs, were randomized to receive 10 mg daily of either isotretinoin or a placebo. The occurrence of skin cancer, compliance and potential treatment toxicity was monitored 6-monthly for 3 years. No significant differences between treatment groups were observed in the 3-year cumulative incidence of BCC or the annual rate of development of new BCCs. However, significant adverse systemic side-effects (in particular, raised serum triglycerides and mucocutaneous toxicity) were seen, even at the low dose administered in this trial (*59*).

Etretinate, BCC/SCC and solar keratoses. While BCCs respond poorly to etretinate therapy (*60*), the suppression of SCCs in four renal transplant patients during 8–13 months of treatment with a dose of 50 mg/day etretinate and also during the following 12 months has been reported (*61*). The treatment of patients with multiple solar keratoses with etretinate has been variably successful (*62, 63* cited in *60*), but the long-term relapse rate and the need for maintenance therapy has not been established.

Topical tretinoin, BCC/SCC and solar keratoses. Tretinoin in ointments or in solution did not appear to be useful in the treatment of small numbers of patients with either BCCs or solar keratoses (*64, 65*). However, Thorne (*66*) has reviewed reports from 31 different centres, in which some 1265 patients with solar keratoses have been evaluated in double-blind studies using 0.05% or 0.1% tretinoin cream for periods of up to 15 months. On the basis of lesion count, and of both the investigators' and patients' assessments, it was deemed that 0.1% tretinoin cream applied for 6 months was most effective in reducing solar keratoses, and the side-effects were said to be well tolerated (*66*). There was a high response rate in the control, vehicle-treated group, although it was suggested that this was because all patients were instructed to apply sunscreens and avoid sun exposure.

Implications for public health policy
Sunscreens
At present, there is no firm evidence on which to base policy regarding the long-term use of sunscreens to prevent skin cancer, since the effectiveness and safety of sunscreen agents applied regularly over periods of years has not yet been established. There is limited evidence that the daily use of a broad-spectrum, high-SPF sunscreen in summer may reduce the development of solar keratoses in populations that are at high risk of actinic skin tumours (*40*). Results of an ongoing trial set in an Australian community (*42*) should provide more information about the preventive potential, and the associated side-effects (as well as the compliance rates among the subjects) of a regimen where adults use a high-protection sunscreen daily for 5 years. It is possible, however, that regular sunscreen use may only be effective against skin cancer if it is commenced in childhood or early adulthood, when initiation of epidermal cells is believed to take place. In view of the possible mutagenicity of certain sunscreen ingredients (*21, 67*), and the uncertain role of UVA as a skin carcinogen (since UVA may not be filtered adequately by many conventional sunscreens), further knowledge is necessary before public policy regarding long-term sunscreen use can be formulated. Moreover, behavioural changes with respect to sun exposure by people using sunscreens could modify the level of achievable protection against skin cancer and solar keratoses. In the meantime, encouragement to use sunscreens to prevent acute erythema (*68*) should assist in the prevention of skin cancer.

Antioxidants
There are no data available to suggest that dietary vitamin supplements offer any population groups protection against skin cancer, including melanoma, or against solar keratoses. However, the potential effectiveness of antioxidants in the reduction of actinic skin lesion has not been fully investigated in humans, and remains a possibility to be considered in appropriate trials, perhaps focusing on intermediate markers, including UV signature mutations in DNA and clinically apparent solar keratoses.

Retinoids
While the toxicity of retinoids in doses that are sufficiently high to be effective against skin cancer and solar keratoses would appear to preclude their widespread use as preventive agents in the general population, considerable side-effects may be tolerated by people who are at very high risk of these tumours (*50*). For example, patients with XP or those with severely sun-damaged skin who persistently develop multiple skin cancers that require regular surgical treatment may benefit from intermittent retinoid therapy.

Conclusion
Chemoprevention may yet prove to be an effective auxiliary measure to include in skin cancer control policies in the future, although it will never replace the need to avoid intense or chronic sun exposure in order to prevent the occurrence of actinic skin disease.

References
1 Marks R, Staples M, Giles GG. Trends in non-melanocytic skin cancer treated in Australia: the second national survey. *Int J Cancer*, 1993, 53:585–590.

2 Miller DL, Weinstock MA. Nonmelanoma skin cancer in the United States: incidence. *J Am Acad Dermatol*, 1994, 30:774–778.

3 Levi F et al. Descriptive epidemiology of skin cancer in the Swiss canton of Vaud. *Int J Cancer*, 1988, 42:811–816.

4 Fidler I. The Biology of skin cancer invasion and metastasis. In: Friedman RJ et al., eds. *Cancer of the skin*. Philadelphia, WB Saunders Co., 1991:3–13.

5 International Agency for Research on Cancer. Solar and ultraviolet radiation. *IARC Monogr Eval Carcinog Risks Humans*. Lyon, IARC, 1992:55.

6 Frost CA, Green AC. Epidemiology of solar keratoses. *Br J Dermatol*, 1994, 131:455–464.

7 Axelrod M, Serafin D, Klitzman B. Ultraviolet light and free radicals: an immunologic theory of epidermal carcinogenesis. *Plast Reconstructive Surgery*, 1990, 86:582–593.

8 Sage E. Distribution and repair of photolesions in DNA: genetic consequences and the role of sequence context. *Photochem Photobiol*, 1993, 57:163–174.

9 Cerutti P. Oxy-radicals and cancer. *Lancet*, 1994, 344:862–836.

10 Ananthaswamy HN, Pierceall WE. Molecular mechanisms of ultraviolet radiation carcinogenesis. *Photochem Photobiol*, 1990, 52:1119–1136.

11 Potten CS et al. DNA damage in UV-irradiated human skin *in vivo*: automated direct measurement by image analysis (thymine dimers) compared with indirect measurement (unscheduled DNA synthesis) and protection by 5-methoxypsoralen. *Int J Radiat Biol*, 1993, 63:313–324.

12 Brash DE et al. A role for sunlight in skin cancer. UV-induced p53 mutations in squamous cell carcinoma. *Proc Natl Acad Sci*, 1991, 88:10124–10128.

13 Rady P et al. p53 mutations in basal cell carcinomas. *Cancer Res*, 1992, 52:3804–3806.

14 Ziegler A et al. Mutation hotspots due to sunlight in p53 gene of nonmelanoma skin cancers. *Proc Natl Acad Sci*, 1993, 90:4216–6220.

15 Kripke ML, Fisher MS. Immunologic parameters of ultraviolet carcinogenesis. *J Natl Cancer Inst*, 1976, 57:211–215.

16 Bouwes Bavinck JN et al. On a possible protective effect of HLA-A11 against skin cancer and keratotic skin lesions in renal transplant recipients. *J Invest Dermatol*, 1991, 97:269–272.

17 Aberer W et al. Langerhans cells as stimulator cells in the murine primary epidermal cell-lymphocyte reaction: alteration by UV-B irradiation. *J Invest Dermatol*, 1982, 79:129–135.

18 Cooper KD et al. Effects of ultraviolet radiation on human epidermal cell alloantigen presentation: initial depression of Langerhans cell-dependent function os followed by the appearance of T6-Dr+cells that enhance epidermal alloantigen presentation. *J Immunol*, 1985, 134:129.

19 Harber LC, DeLeo VA, Prystowsky JH. Intrinsic and extrinsic photoprotection against UVB and UVA radiation. In: Lowe NJ, ed. *Physician's guide to sunscreens*. New York, Marcel Dekker, 1991:141–160.

20 Pathak MA. Topical and systemic approaches for the prevention of acute and chronic sun-induced skin reactions. *Dermatol Clinics*, 1986, 4:321–334.

21 Young AR. 5-methoxypsoralen-containing sunscreens. In: Lowe NJ, ed. *Physician's guide to sunscreens*. New York, Marcel Dekker, 1991:81–93.

22 Freeman SE, Ley KD. Sunscreen protection against UV-induced pyrimidine dimers in DNA of human skin in situ. *Photodermatol*, 1988, 5:243–247.

23 Young AR, Gibbs NK, Magnus IA. Modification of 5-methoxypsoralen phototumorigenesis by UVB sunscreens: a statistical and histologic study in the hairless albino mouse. *J Invest Dermatol*, 1987, 89:611–617.

24 Chadwick CA et al. The time of onset and duration of 5-methoxypsoralen photochemoprotection from UVR-induced DNA damage in human skin. *Br J Dermatol*, 1994, 131:483–494.

25 Kligman LH, Akin FJ, Kligman AM. Sunscreens prevent ultraviolet photocarcinogenesis. *J Am Acad Dermatol*, 1980, 3:30–35.

26 Wulf HC et al. Sunscreens for delay of ultraviolet induction of skin tumours. *J Am Acad Dermatol*, 1982, 7:194–202.

27 Forbes PD et al. Inhibition of ultraviolet radiation-induced skin tumors in hairless mice by topical application of the sunscreen 2-ethyl hexyl-p-methoxycinnamate. *J Toxicol: Cut & Ocular Toxicol*, 1989, 8:209–226.

28 Flindt-Hansen H, Thune P, Eeg-Larsen T. The effect of short-term application of PABA on photocarcinogenesis. *Acta Derm Venereol*, 1990, 70:72–75.

29 Bissett DL et al. Time-dependent decrease in sunscreen protection against chronic photodamage in UVB-irradiated hairless mouse skin. *J Photochem Photobiol*, 1991, 9:323–334.

30 Wolf P, Donawho CK, Kripke ML. Effect of sunscreens on UV radiation-induced enhancement of melanoma growth in mice. *J Nat Cancer Inst*, 1994, 86:99–105.

31 Garland CF, Garland FC, Gorham ED. Rising trends in melanoma. A hypothesis concerning sunscreen effectiveness. *Ann Epidemiol*, 1993, 3:103–110.

32 Santamaria L et al. Chemoprevention of indirect and direct chemical carcinogenesis by carotenoids as oxygen radical quenchers. *Ann NY Acad Sci*, 1988, 534:584–96.

33 Fryer MJ. Evidence for the photoprotective effects of vitamin E. *Photochem Photobiol*, 1993, 58:304–313.

34 van Poppel G. Carotenoids and cancer: an update with emphasis on human intervention studies. *Eur J Cancer*, 1993, 29:1335–1344.

35 Fuller CJ et al. Effect of β-carotene supplementation on photosuppression of delayed-type hypersensitivity in normal young men. *Am J Clin Nutr*, 1992, 56:684–690.

36 Bendich A. Physiological role of antioxidants in the immune system. J *Dairy Sci*, 1993, 76:2789–2794.

37 Kwa R, Campana K, Moy RL. Biology of cutaneous squamous cell carcinoma. *J Am Acad Dermatol*, 1992, 26:1–26.

38 Malkovsky M et al. Enhancement of specific anti-tumor immunity in mice fed a diet enriched in vitamin A acetate. *Proc Natl Acad Sci*, 1983, 80:6322–6326.

39 Kligman LH. Photoaging manifestations, prevention, and treatment. *Dermatol Clin*, 1986, 4:517.

40 Thompson SC, Jolley D, Marks R. Reduction of solar keratoses by regular sunscreen use. *N Eng J Med*, 1993, 329:1147–1151.

41 Foley P et al. The frequency of reactions to sunscreens: results of a longitudinal population-based study on the regular use of sunscreens in Australia. *Br J Dermatol*, 1993, 128:857–863.

42 Green A et al. and the Nambour Prevention Study Group. Nambour Skin Cancer and Actinic Eye Disease Prevention Trial: Design and Baseline Characteristics of Participants. *Controlled Clin Trials*, 1994, 15:512–522.

43 Kune GA et al. Diet, alcohol, smoking, serum β-carotene, and vitamin A in male nonmelanocytic skin cancer patients and controls. *Nutr Cancer*, 1992, 18:237–244.

44 Shekelle RB et al. Dietary vitamin A and risk of cancer in the Western Electric Study. *Lancet*, 1981, 2:1186–1190.

45 Wald N et al. Serum beta-carotene and subsequent risk of cancer. *Br J Cancer*, 1988, 57:428–435.

46 Comstock GW, Bush TL, Helzlsouer K. Serum retinol, beta-carotene, vitamin E and selenium as related to subsequent cancer of specific sites. *Am J Epidemiol*, 1992, 135:115–21.

47 Hunter DJ et al. Diet and risk of basal cell carcinoma of the skin in prospective cohort of women. Ann Epidemiol, 1992, 2:231–239.

48 Greenberg ER et al. and the Skin Cancer Prevention Group. The skin cancer prevention study: design of a clinical trial of beta-carotene among persons at high risk for nonmelanoma skin cancer. *Controlled Clin Trials*, 1989, 10:153–166.

49 Greenberg ER et al. and the Skin Cancer Prevention Group. A clinical trial of beta carotene to prevent basal-cell and squamous-cell cancers of the skin. *N Engl J Med*, 1990, 323:789–95.

50 Meyskens FL. Coming of age – the chemoprevention of cancer. *New Eng J Med*, 1990, 323:825–827.

51 Karagas MR et al. Risk of subsequent basal cell carcinoma and squamous cell carcinoma of the skin among patients with prior skin cancer. *JAMA*, 1992, 267:3305–3310.

52 Stryker WS et al. Diet, plasma levels of beta-carotene and alpha-tocopherol, and risk of malignant melanoma. *Am J Epidemiol*, 1990, 131:597–611.

53 Bain C et al. Diet and melanoma. An exploratory case–control study. *Ann Epidemiol*, 1993, 3:235–238.

54 Knekt P et al. Serum micronutrients and risk of cancer of low incidence in Finland. *Am J Epidemiol*, 1991, 134:356–61.

55 Kraemer KH et al. Prevention of skin cancer in xeroderma pigmentosum with the use of oral isotretinoin. *N Eng J Med*, 1988, 318:1633–1637.

56 Kraemer KH, DiGiovanna JJ, Peck GL. Chemoprevention of skin cancer in xeroderma pigmentosum. *J Dermatol*, 1992, 19:715–718.

57 Peck GL. Long-term retinoid therapy is needed for maintenance of cancer chemopreventive effect. *Dermatologica*, 1987, 175:138–144.

58 Tangrea JA et al. Long-term therapy with low-dose isotretinoin for prevention of basal cell carcinoma: a multicenter clinical trial. *J Nat Cancer Inst*, 1992, 84:328–332.

59 Tangrea JA et al. for the Isotretinoin-Basal Cell Carcinoma Study Group. Clinical and laboratory adverse effects associated with long-term, low-dose isotretinoin: Incidence and risk factors. *Cancer Epidemiol Biomarkers Prevent*, 1993, 2:375–380.

60 Peck GL. Topical tretinoin in actinic keratosis and basal cell carcinoma. *J Am Acad Dermatol*, 1986, 15:829–835.

61 Kelly JW et al. Retinoids to prevent skin cancer in organ transplant recipients. *Lancet*, 1991, 338:1407.

62 Moriaty M, Dunn J, Darragh A. Etretinate in the treatment of actinic keratosis. *Lancet*, 1982, 1:364–365.

63 Berretti B, Grupper C. Cutaneous neoplasia and etretinate. In Cunliffe WJ, Miller AJ, eds. *Retinoid therapy*. Lancaster, MTP Press, 1984:187–194.

64 Bollag W, Ott F. Vitamin A in benign and malignant epithelial tumours of the skin. *Acta Derm Venerol (Suppl)*, 1975, 74:163–166

65 Robinson TA, Kligman AM: Treatment of solar keratoses with retinoic acid and 4-fluorouracil. *Br J Dermatol*, 1975, 92:703–706.

66 Thorne EG. Long-term clinical experience with a topical retinoid. *Br J Dermatol*, 1992, 127:31–36.

67 Knowland J et al. Sunlight-induced mutagenicity of a common sunscreen ingredient. *Fed Europe Biochem Societies*, 1993, 324:309–313.

68 Drolet BA, Connor MJ. Sunscreens and the prevention of ultraviolet radiation-induced skin cancer. *J Dermatol Surg Oncol*, 1992, 18:571–576.

A. Green
Queensland Institute of Medical Research,
P.O. Royal Brisbane Hospital, Queensland 4029,
Australia

Ethical issues of intervention trials in cancer

H. Sancho-Garnier* and R. Joseph

The objective of cancer prevention is either a reduction in the incidence of the disease, through direct action against its causes, or a reduction of its morbidity and mortality.

Chemoprevention trials are not innocuous. They involve healthy subjects. As a consequence, careful ethical consideration must be given to such programmes. In particular, calculating the risk–benefit ratio must take into account not only the physical but also the mental and social well-being of people whose lives will be 'medicalized' as a result of such intervention. The primacy of collective benefit over individual interest demands that preventive intervention be based on voluntary informed consent of the target population. The numerous consequences of the extrapolation of results of chemoprevention trials to the general population must be considered. Finally, the classical contract between patient and doctor is altered in this novel situation. The promotion of research into the psychological and social consequences of chemoprevention of cancer is essential.

Ethical issues

Cancer prevention aims to produce either a reduction in the incidence of the disease, through direct action against its causes, or a reduction of its morbidity and mortality, by attacking the process leading to clinical expression of the cancer (1).

Prevention strategies include :

- elimination or reduction of exposure to risk factors, e.g. smoking cessation strategies;
- elimination of the effect of these exposures by the use of protective factors, e.g. vaccination, diet;
- treatment of precancerous lesions which have a high probability of evolution into cancer, e.g. colon polyps, cervical dysplasia;
- screening and treatment of cancers at a stage of maximum curability, e.g. breast cancer.

The first type of action uses only public information, education and legislative methods. All the other strategies include diagnostic and therapeutic medical procedures.

*Correspondence: H. Sancho-Garnier, Hôpital G, Doumergue CHU, Nîmes 3000, France.

Preventive medicine is not innocuous, particularly when such actions are based on medical interventions (2). Preventive efforts should not lead to an impairment of the physical, mental or social well-being of the individual concerned. Furthermore, prevention generally applies to healthy subjects, i.e. those not needing medical care and for whom, in the majority of cases, there will be no direct benefit. Because of the haphazard and delayed nature of the benefits of intervention trials, the risk–benefit ratio of such actions must take into account not only their physical effects but also their psychological and social consequences.

The undesirable effects of preventive interventions are often poorly recognized. The attendant risks are run by the entire healthy population, while the target disease only affects a (usually small) portion of the individuals constituting this population. Even if the intervention brings a slight advantage to a reasonably large number of subjects, a significant risk of undesirable effects, even for a minority of them, is difficult to accept. An intervention trial should not be undertaken unless the expected benefits outweigh the potential risks

Benefits are represented by a decrease in incidence and/or mortality rates of a disease, which may or may not be associated with an improvement in the quality of life. Interventions trials should be conducted under conditions that are most likely to give reliable results, e.g. scientific rationale, correct methodology, careful choice of target population, correct treatment doses and duration, good quality control, etc. Unless these criteria are met the interventions must be considered unethical.

Potential ill-effects are numerous and varied. On the one hand, any toxicity of preventive agents is usually carefully observed and documented, even when unexpected, while on the other hand, the potential psychological and social consequences, such as those described below, are generally ignored.

Taking medication daily and/or submitting to repeated testing may lead healthy subjects to consider themselves as potentially or actually ill, or at least to be constantly conscious of the possibility of getting cancer. Preventive intervention leads to false hopes for those who will get the disease despite compliance with the suggested programme. As a result, these patients and their relatives may experience serious disillusionment with standard medicine (3). Study subjects who forget to take their medication or who drop out of a trial prematurely could develop chronic anxiety as to the possible risks of their behaviour.

Development of cancer in patients who decline to participate in, or who do not comply with, chemoprevention trials may engender profound guilt.

Initiation of large-scale trials is often followed by major media coverage. This may lead a proportion of the population to self-prescribe the medication involved in the trial before any efficacy has been proven. Such publicity may also engender mass cancerophobia.

Ethical reflection necessitates going beyond the evaluation of the risk–benefit ratio of an intervention, as already advocated by many authors (4) in the 1970s. The probability of benefit to the individual is low, and the benefit is uncertain (random) and late. The individual participant must therefore accept the primacy of collective benefit over individual interest. These considerations thus necessitate that this type of intervention be based on voluntary informed consent of the target population. It is in this context, where the interest of the research itself and the interest of the subjects almost inevitably come into confrontation, that the principle of informed consent is most important.

One must also consider the consequences of extrapolating results of chemoprevention trials to the general population (5). If the results are in favour of chemoprevention, will this type of intervention be applicable to millions of people? For example, is it imaginable that a large part of the population will swallow a handful of various medications (vitamins, microelements, ASA, hormones, etc.) every day for the rest of their lives to avoid various illnesses? Where will we stop? Furthermore, will it be possible with such a mixture of agents to determine the contribution of each to the desired effect or to predict toxic interactions? Will toxicities, whose low frequencies are acceptable in the context of a clinical trial, become unacceptable

given the large denominator of the general population? Will not the economic cost of such intervention be prohibitive.

Finally, the ethical problems inherent in intervention trials cannot be resolved in the framework of the classical contract between patient and doctor. Traditionally, the patient comes to the physician seeking care. On the other hand, in chemoprevention it is the physician who proposes the intervention. This basic difference from usual medical practice demands that, before instituting such trials, the collective rather than the individual consequences of the trial should be seriously considered.

Measurement of the effects of preventive interventions on the lifestyle and mental health of the population subjected to them necessitates the development of specific tools adapted to such situations. The promotion of future research in this area is essential.

References

1 Buiatti E. *Intervention trials of cancer prevention: results and new research programmes.* International Agency for Research on Cancer, Lyon, (IARC Technical Report No. 18). 1994.

2 Maheu E. La prévention entre responsabilité et coercition. In: *Idéologies de la prévention.* Revue AGORA - Ethique Médecine, Société, 30, 1994: 3–7.

3 Bouvier P et al. Aspects éthiques du dépistage: réflexions à partir de l'exemple du cancer du sein. Cahier médico-sociaux. *Ed Médecine et Hygiène*, 1994, 38:1.

4 Jeanneret O, Raymond L. Aspects éthiques des études d'intervention. *Rev Epidem et Santé Publ*, 1981, 129:269–279.

5 Lazar P. Vaut il toujours mieux prévenir que guérir? *La revue du praticien*, 1994, 44:2533–2534.

H. Sancho-Garnier
Hôpital G, Doumergue CHU, Nîmes 3000, France

R. Joseph
Medical College of Pennsylvania, Philadelphia, PA 19129, USA

Behavioural intervention versus chemoprevention

M. Henderson*, B. Thompson and A. Kristal

To be effective on a population level, cancer control programmes must be comprehensive and have the capacity to prevent cancer. A fundamental public health principle is that the modification of risk behaviours has a much wider application than does the treatment of the consequences of those behaviours. Chemoprevention efforts, while having some public health implications, are somewhat limited in their application. Behavioural interventions, on the other hand, have the potential to change risk behaviour before a chemopreventive agent is needed. Despite the appeal of behavioural intervention trials, a number of important issues remain to be addressed before they can be implemented. One basic issue is the reliance of behavioural trials on the strategies, methods and procedures of randomized clinical (therapeutic) trials, and on the empirical and statistical data upon which these trials are based. This information does not always meet the needs of behavioural intervention studies. In this paper, we discuss the differences in the applications of behavioural and chemoprevention trials, the goals of behavioural intervention trials, and areas where more information is needed to fully understand such trials.

Introduction

To be effective at the population level, cancer control programmes must be comprehensive and have the capacity to prevent cancer. A fundamental, related public health principle is that modification of risk behaviours themselves has a much wider application than does the treatment of the consequences of those behaviours. Although some researchers believe that chemopreventive agents have potential for public health applications, others hold that for reasons of safety and cost the use of most chemopreventive agents should be limited to persons at very high risk. Only a few potential chemopreventive agents have demonstrated acceptability and safety. Recent results from the Finnish study of β-carotene and vitamin E, however, indicate that

*Correspondence: M. Henderson, Cancer Prevention Research Program, Fred Hutchinson Cancer Research Center, 1124 Columbia, MP-702, Seattle, WA 98104, USA.

the efficacy and safety of even the most benign-seeming chemoprevention therapy is not assured.

Behavioural interventions have important advantages for population-level prevention. They carry a low risk of side-effects, and these side-effects tend to be positive (e.g. self-efficacy and well-being). There is some evidence that individuals prefer taking pills to changing their behaviour, as demonstrated by the 40% of United States citizens who report taking vitamins regularly (1); however, people generally report that they would rather change behaviour than take pills. In a survey of Washington State residents by random digit dialling, for example, 83% of both male and female respondents reported that they would prefer to prevent cancer by eating a vegetable at lunch and dinner each day, as compared with 14% who said they would prefer taking a pill (2). A similar preference for lifestyle change rather than treatment was found in a community-wide survey of women aged 65–75 years; 90.8% said they would prefer to make a major change in their diet than to take a pill daily to prevent disease (3).

In this paper we describe some of the goals of behavioural intervention trials and areas where more information is needed in order to utilize their advantages fully. We will also discuss some differences between the attributes of behavioural intervention and chemoprevention trials, as an indication of the roles which each can play in cancer control. Some of the features of lifestyle modification trials (their design, evaluation and methodology) lead us to the conclusion that definitive trials of the effectiveness of behavioural intervention cannot be conducted until there has been more extensive and in-depth research on relevant models, strategies and tools. For purposes of clarity, this discussion is limited to modification of exposure-related lifestyle behaviours that have the potential for primary prevention. We focus on community-wide intervention, arguing that individual behavioural interventions are unlikely to have much of a public health impact. Current candidates for intervention include cigarette smoking, high fat, low fruit and vegetable dietary patterns, and exposure to the sun.

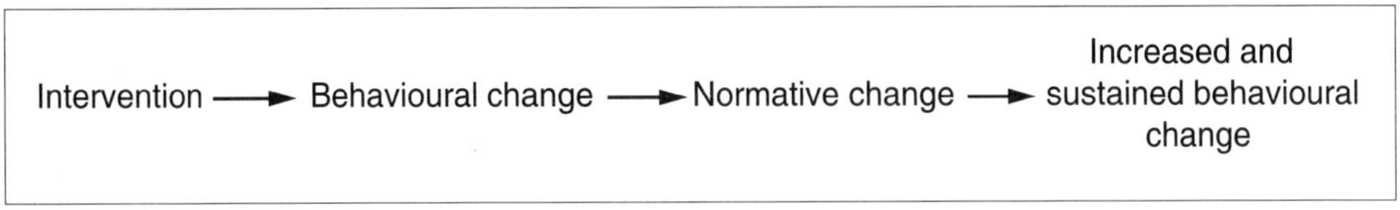

Intervention ⟶ Behavioural change ⟶ Normative change ⟶ Increased and sustained behavioural change

Fig 1. Successful community-wide intervention.

Behavioural interventions

Interventions to modify behaviour can be roughly classified into three groups, according to their goals: behaviours to modify lifestyles related to exposure (4, 5, 6, 7, 8), behaviours to modify the use of screening tests (9, 10), and behaviours to modify compliance with treatment protocols and adherence to prescribed regimens (11). In terms of cancer outcomes, the first would lead to changes in cancer incidence, the second would lead to changes in the rates of early detection of cancer and the distribution of its stages at diagnosis, and the third would lead to changes in case fatality. Only the first – modification in lifestyle exposures – results in primary prevention. Modification of the use of screening procedures can affect population-wide rates of mortality, but not incidence. Screening procedures can be more intensely applied to subgroups at high risk (for reasons of costs and safety), and may thus have even less chance of affecting population-level mortality. Treatment and prescribed regimens are rarely applicable to the public at large, and are consequently unlikely to bring about improvements in any population-wide measurements of the impact of cancer.

It has been well argued that a relatively small average population-wide change in a cancer-related behaviour can lead to a measurable improvement in cancer incidence and prevalence (12, 13, 14). This is especially true if lifestyle changes are well diffused through all groups in the population at risk, both volunteers and non-volunteers for intervention (12, 13). As will be discussed shortly, current theoretical approaches to behaviour focus on the natural history of behaviour changes; that is, they attempt to work within the process of behaviour change rather than interrupting it with a sudden new demand. Most of the current public health and diffusion models accommodate the need to emphasize changes that are congruent with the natural history of specific human behaviours, although these models have yet to be rigorously tested. One of the major differences between change in motivated individuals and change on a community-wide or population-wide level is the feedback and input from the community as a social organization. As Fig. 1 indicates, an intervention which is successful at the community level can be expected to increase over the years subsequent to the intervention; this is based on the belief that change that is sufficiently prevalent to influence community health will also be widespread enough to influence community norms in terms of the behaviour itself (15, 16, 17). In other words, the intervention process itself will induce changes in normative values, which in turn will lead to more and greater changes in the targeted lifestyle (18). This belief that a successful community intervention becomes prolonged and intensified through its own dynamic process increases confidence that it may also result in a sustained change which will influence disease rates in more than one generation. However, more research is still needed to examine this assumption, particularly on interventions simple enough to be used by everyone but intensive enough to initiate long-lasting change.

Experience with behavioural interventions for cancer prevention

There is more accumulated experience with interventions to modify cigarette smoking and other tobacco use behaviours than with interventions to modify any other lifestyle that exposes large numbers of the general public to carcinogens (5, 7). Conceptually, this should be an easy behaviour to change, because the relationship between tobacco use and lung cancer is extremely strong – in developed countries, approximately 91% of lung cancers in men and 62% in women are caused by smoking (19). Evidence of the benefit of quitting is so unequivocal that a change in smoking behaviour, from smoker to non-smoker, has become the principal measure of successful intervention.

Consequently, the design of interventions to prevent children and adolescents from taking up smoking, and to motivate and help smokers of all ages to quit smoking have been based on state of the art understanding of the natural history of changes in cigarette smoking behaviour (20, 21, 22). These interventions have been relatively successful in bringing about the planned, short-term changes in individuals included in the studies (23, 24, 25). The success of these trials in many different populations encouraged investigators in the USA to move ahead with research to bring about changes in the smoking behaviour of entire communities (26, 27).

Attempts to modify other disease-related behaviours in individuals have been less successful. The modest results of trials of dietary modifications to lower blood cholesterol and body mass among individual high-risk participants may be in part due to the poor congruence of intervention and its concomitant measure of success, and the investigators' uncertainty in building an intervention around a model of the natural history of a behaviour when the strength of the association between that behaviour and the desired biological effect is unknown (28). For example, controversy exists as to the amount of reduction in serum cholesterol that can be achieved by modifying dietary patterns (29, 30, 31). Similarly, caloric intake by itself is not a good indicator of body weight (32, 33, 34). More research is needed in these areas.

Common theoretical underpinnings of behavioural change can be identified regardless of the particular behaviour targeted. The current theoretical framework for cigarette smoking interventions provides a good example: it suggests that a range of interventions is needed which coincides with a number of more or less distinct but transitional stages in the spectrum of the behaviour's natural history (22, 35). The smokers themselves must have some control over the intervention process; however, a supportive environment is essential to sustain the new behaviour (35). A continuing sense of individual self-confidence in the ability to manage a new behavioural change also appears to play a role in the maintenance of the new behaviour (35, 36, 37). The complexity of translating this paradigm – stage-matched interventions; individuals participating in the management of their own behavioural change; an encouraging social environment – becomes amplified several times over when it is put

into the context of community intervention. In a cost-effective community intervention, the target individuals must be all the members of the community – e.g. both smokers who have and smokers who have never thought of quitting, non-smokers who have never thought about helping smokers to change their lifestyles, and all those individuals who will work together towards a smoke-free environment. The relationship between the supportiveness of a community's social environment for a new behaviour and the long-term results of community intervention has led some investigators to consider the development of such a social environment to be an integral part of the design of a trial, if not of the intervention itself. An example is seen in the tobacco control field, where funded projects, such as the American Stop Smoking Intervention Study (ASSIST) and the Robert Wood Johnson 'Smokeless States Initiative', consider the implementation of public policies around tobacco taxation, access and advertisement to be the intervention of choice (27, 38).

Changes in individual health-related behaviours have been described both empirically and on a theoretical basis. In most cases, the behavioural change interventions were not carried out in the context of a supportive social environment. The intervention processes found to be successful in such studies can be linked to different theoretical constructs if they are embedded in a more inclusive context. For example, analyses of the trends of long-lasting change in eating patterns of women in a dietary intervention trial showed that women made a large change in their daily fat consumption as soon as they were given the tools to make and measure that change, and that the extent of their long-term (1.5–5 years) changes in fat consumption depended upon the extent of the initial change (39, 40). The initial change, whether small or large, was sustained, and neither increased nor decreased over time (39). This finding is analogous to a situation in which 'cold turkey quitters' (those who withdraw from smoking abruptly) achieve as much success in abstaining from the use of tobacco products as quitters who gradually reduce their tobacco consumption (41). These individual processes of change, however, generally occur in the absence of environmental support. It may be that such support would provide an added boost to continue the trend in reduction in fat consumption.

One of the great advantages of intervening to modify the natural history of a behaviour, rather than designing a trial which prescribes an agent to interrupt the natural history of a specific disease, is that the change in behaviour can influence more than one disease process. Successful modification of cigarette smoking, for example, should result in a reduction in incidence rates of some other cancers and in reductions in death rates from chronic lung and coronary heart disease (7, 42, 43). Several cancer-related lifestyles, such as eating patterns, are similarly associated with the risks of other diseases, and changes in these lifestyles should provide greater and more lasting health benefits than would interventions designed simply to modify the natural history of a specific disease (6, 44, 45).

Attributes of behavioural intervention and chemoprevention trials

In the design of a community-wide cancer prevention programme, primary prevention through lifestyle modification contrasts with, but is complementary to, chemoprevention. This can be illustrated by examining some attributes of the two approaches.

- The calculated cost of a life saved through reduction of cancer incidence is low with behavioural intervention and high with chemoprevention. In calculating the costs per life saved, pre-screening for high risk, assessment of eligibility, safety monitoring and follow-up must be included among the necessary costs of chemoprevention.
- Behavioural interventions are applicable to virtually all the people in a community, whereas chemoprevention is almost always limited to those at high risk. Behavioural intervention creates a modest reduction in the risks of an entire population which can potentially lead to an improvement in the public's health. Successful chemoprevention in any population may prove to be capable of bringing about a relatively large reduction in the risk of a limited number of high-risk individuals, but the sum of these benefits may be rather modest, when measured as disease rates in the whole population.
- Behavioural intervention reduces exposure to toxic agents (in this case carcinogenic), whereas chemoprevention contains tissue damage after exposure to these agents has occurred.

- Since it changes community norms in terms of a more favourable distribution of exposures and risks, behavioural intervention protects future generations. Chemoprevention has no influence at all on the exposure of future cohorts.
- Only positive side-effects have been documented in association with behavioural interventions to date (e.g. increased feelings of self-efficacy and well-being), while the side-effects of chemoprevention are usually negative, and may be difficult to determine except in the case of a very large trial which continues follow-up for many years.
- Behavioural interventions with the potential for community-wide influence often have comprehensive effects, with an impact upon the natural history of several different malignancies (for example, cigarette smoking). Chemoprevention is more likely to be specific to one aetiological pathway or to one malignant tumour.
- Behavioural intervention can be applied (and its benefits achieved) even when causal mechanisms are not understood. Implementation of chemoprevention requires some understanding of the biology and aetiology of the target cancer.

Issues for behavioural research

In terms of methodology, chemoprevention trials depend heavily on the strategies, methods and procedures of randomized trials, and on the statistical theory upon which their principles are based. These data frequently do not meet the needs of investigators responsible for behavioural intervention. As a result, a more extensive development of models, strategies and tools is needed for trials of the effectiveness of behavioural interventions.

Behavioural intervention research rests upon an extensive theoretical base. Both the behavioural interventions themselves and the community intervention approach are, and should be, theory-driven. Although the expected performance of theoretically derived paradigms for the design and evaluation of these trials should be quantified through modelling research, this is rarely done. Quantification of any and all well understood processes of behavioural change is urgently needed.

Community trials involve the application of interventions known to be efficacious. Any preceding trials that evaluated efficacy will have had very similar parameters to a chemoprevention or clinical trial, using the same overarching principles and procedures, and will have been carried out among randomized individuals who are largely self-selected. There has been a less than complete understanding and appreciation that the next step – the population-based trial using the proven behavioural intervention – is unique to prevention and does not yet have a tried and tested set of theoretically derived or empirically developed strategies and methods for either intervention or research. Some methodological findings from clinical trials among consenting patients or participants have direct implications for population-based trials, and can also be used to highlight the need for much more research to be directed towards the development of a sound methodological base for community-wide or population-wide trials of effectiveness.

A major limitation of efficacy trials is that they are often conducted among motivated participants and under the best of circumstances. Very small proportions of the defined population at risk volunteer for, or become enrolled in, a trial. Estimates of recruits to prevention trials are of the order of one to five people per thousand at risk (46). Thus, it is not only the hard-to-reach groups in the at-risk population who do not participate in the usual intervention research, but also the majority of its easy-to-reach groups. Studies among smokers, for example, have consistently shown that only 1–10% of active smokers join any smoking cessation research activities (24, 47). Smoking cessation interventions are therefore being tested among a self-selected small proportion of the smokers who are ready to quit, and ignore the larger pool of smokers. On the whole, no rigorous evaluation of smoking interventions directed at volunteers can be expected to include such subgroups as blue collar, minority and adolescent smokers, who are all recognized as being hard to reach (5).

Similarly, only 1–5% of the population at risk takes part in activities related to dietary change (46). Thus, currently available tools for changing individual dietary patterns have been evaluated in populations that under-represent men and have almost never included individuals from hard-to-reach, minority or disadvantaged groups – the groups that are probably most in need of dietary change. The use of motivated volunteers leads to a subset of individuals who are most likely to make a behavioural change.

The widest possible recruitment is clearly a research strategy which must be developed for behavioural intervention research that is to be widely applicable. There are other equally urgent and important needs, which begin with the interventions themselves. Behavioural interventions must be simple and cheap enough to be adopted and managed by everyone in the population, and sufficiently intensive to bring about changes that are effective and long-lasting. Based on current theory, there must be a number of complementary interventions, or the intervention plan must call for sequences of complementary interventions. Given that the expected changes will take time to be taken up, to spread to other individuals and groups, and to intensify, it is very difficult to know the appropriate intervals at which outcomes should be measured.

It is not known why some behavioural changes persist, or for how long they may do so. Since exposure to carcinogens lasts for many years before cancer develops, lifestyle modifications must persist for more than a year or two to be effective in prevention. At the very least, the initial behavioural change has to persist (and better yet, to increase) in individuals over the years after the intervention itself is completed. For example, a study directed at women which targeted low-fat diets showed that women maintained their dietary change (48). Furthermore, the women's husbands also adopted the dietary change, providing support for the notion that environmental change has an impact on behaviour (49).

Other well recognized issues in the statistical design of studies of community intervention include the relative advantages of sequential cross-sectional versus cohort outcome measures (50, 51), the relative advantages of pairing communities prior to randomization (52, 53), and the extent to which an intervention community that develops a successful population-wide organization can define its own process of intervention (54). This latter feature contrasts with the axiom of clinical trials of efficacy, where standardized formulations and doses of experimental drugs are *de rigueur*. If measurements of biological availability and pharmacokinetic profiles were used as the standards in these trials, and prescribed dosages and instructions for use to achieve these levels were allowed to vary, they would be more analogous to the community intervention trial model, in which the intensity and frequency of the intervention is prescribed on the community level, although not on the individual level.

Unfortunately, there has been no research carried out to provide the behavioural equivalent to the biomedical body of knowledge about bioequivalency and pharmacokinetics. What is usually described as process research in human behavioural change has been poorly supported in the past and has rarely, if ever, been quantified beyond the individual. Understanding the mechanisms by which human behaviour is changed in both the short and long term is as important as understanding the mechanisms by which any other body function is changed; it must thus be amenable to some form of quantification. A simple example already mentioned is the lack of knowledge of how long an intervention needs to be applied and left in place in order to bring about long-lasting change; whether the ratio of intensity and duration of the application of an intervention is important in that decision; and the extent to which quantification of one or both of these parameters determines the appropriate timing of the outcome measures.

The rate at which the social environment (and not just the individual) changes is another important determinant of the length of time that should pass before long-lasting change can be measured. Have any trials to date intervened over a long enough period to ensure that the social environment is sufficiently supportive? Have any trials waited for the combined effects of diffusion and changes in norms to have their full impact before they made their outcome measurements?

Another important research question is whether a trial can capitalize on a secular trend in order to cut short the length of time needed to build up an environment that is supportive enough to sustain the changed target behaviour. At what rate of increase in the secular trend do the disadvantages of an experimental trial outweigh the advantages? For example, a community smoking prevention trial that does not take advantage of a secular trend to increase restrictive policies governing youth access to tobacco products may find itself falling behind comparison communities that work actively to implement such policies. In such a situation, maintaining an intervention protocol that was written before the secular trend developed may actually impede the attainment of a trial-wide objective to prevent the onset of tobacco use among young people. A supportive environment is a key element in terms of sustaining as well as creating behavioural change, so a certain degree of increase in a secular trend may well maximize the long-lasting outcomes in an effectiveness trial, and more than offset any contamination of the comparison communities by that trend; however, the balance has to be quantified and measured.

Conclusion

If it is successful, community intervention should be the most cost-effective, safe and long-lasting approach to cancer control. It would provide the ideal background and context for the practice of chemoprevention, for risk assessment and for early detection and treatment. Unfortunately, research to date has been inadequate to demonstrate the full potential of behavioural intervention in terms of long-lasting behavioural or biological outcomes.

The aetiological associations between behaviour and cancer risk are complex and multifactorial. Thus, although chemopreventive agents may prove effective in the prevention of some specific cancers, it is unlikely that they will address all the negative consequences of lifestyle exposures. Even though the biomedical scientific community tends to be pessimistic about being able to bring about widespread changes in lifestyle behaviours such as smoking and eating patterns, it seems even less likely that we will be able to manufacture a safe cigarette or produce an elixir of chemopreventive agents that will counteract the biological consequences of smoking and eating behaviours.

In this paper, we have argued that behavioural intervention can and should play a major role in cancer prevention and control; that community intervention and some of its research requirements are unique to prevention research; that the state of the art of this research is too rudimentary to be able to test the full potential of behavioural intervention; and that there is some urgency in the need to support and carry out the necessary methodological research so that other major community-wide behavioural intervention trials that are proposed and funded can maximize the opportunity of achieving positive results.

References

1 Bender MM et al. Trends in prevalence and magnitude of vitamin and mineral supplement usage and correlation with health status. *J Am Diet Assoc*, 1992, 92:1096–1101.

2 Kristal AR et al. The effects of enhanced calling efforts in random digit dial surveys on response rates, population-level estimates of health behavior, and costs. *Pub Health Rep*, 1993, 108:372–380.

3 Urban N. The Community Mammography Project. Seattle, WA, Fred Hutchinson Cancer Research Center, 1993.

4 National Research Council. Diet and Health: Implications for Reducing Chronic Disease Risk. *Report of the Committee on Diet and Health, Food and Nutrition Board, Commission on Life Sciences.* Washington, DC, National Academy Press, 1989.

5 US Department of Health and Human Services. *Reducing the health consequences of smoking: 25 years of progress. A report of the Surgeon General.* Washington, DC, US Government Printing Office, 1989 (DHHS Publ. No. CDC 89–8411).

6 US Department of Health and Human Services. *Healthy people 2000.* Washington, DC, US Government Printing Office, 1990 (DHHS Publ. No. PHS 91–50212).

7 US Department of Health and Human Services. *The health benefits of smoking cessation. A report of the Surgeon General.* Washington, DC, US Government Printing Office, 1990 (DHHS Publ. No. CDC 90–8416).

8 Steinmetz K, Potter JD. A review of vegetables, fruit, and cancer I *Epidemiology: Cancer Causes and Control,* 1991, 2:325–357.

9 Miller AB et al., eds. *Cancer screening.* Cambridge, UK, Cambridge University Press, 1991.

10 White E, Urban N, Taylor V. Mammography utilization, public health impact, and cost-effectiveness in the United States. *Ann Rev Public Health,* 1993, 14:605–633.

11 Sackett DL, Haynes RB. *Compliance with therapeutic regimes.* Baltimore, The Johns Hopkins University Press, 1976.

12 Rose G. Sick individuals and sick populations. *Int J Epidemiol,* 1985, 14:32–38.

13 Rose G. Future of disease prevention: British perspective on the US preventive services task force guidelines. *J Gen Intern Med,* 1990, 5:S123–S128.

14 Kristal AR. Nutritional intervention: how can we meet the 'Healthy People 2000' goals? *Med Exerc Nutr Health,* 1993, 2:3–4.

15 Farquhar J. The community-based model of life style intervention trials. *Am J Epidemiol,* 1978, 108:103–111.

16 Green LW, Raeburn J. Contemporary developments in health promotion: definitions and challenges. In: Bracht N, ed. *Health promotion at the community level.* Newbury Park, CA, Sage Publications, 1990:29–44.

17 Thompson B, Kinne S. Social change theory: applications to community health. In: Bracht N, ed. *Health promotion at the community level.* Newberry Park, CA, Sage Publications, 1990:45–65.

18 Thompson B et al. Principles of community organization and partnership for smoking cessation in the Community Intervention Trial for Smoking Cessation (COMMIT). *Int Q Commun Health Educ,* 1991, 11:187–203.

19 Parkin DM et al. At least one in seven cases of cancer is caused by smoking: global estimates for 1985. *Int J Cancer,* 1994, 59:494–504.

20 Prochaska JO, DiClemente C. Self change processes, self-efficacy and decisional balance across five stages of smoking cessation. *Prog Clin Biol Res,* 1984, 51:390–395.

21 Prochaska JO, DiClemente CC. Predicting change in smoking status for self-changers. *Addict Behav,* 1985, 10:395–406.

22 Prochaska JO. Patterns of change in smoking behavior. *Health Psychol,* 1986, 5:97–98.

23 Janz NK et al. Evaluation of a miminal-contact smoking cessation intervention in an outpatient setting. *Am J Public Health,* 1987, 77:805–809.

24 Fisher KJ, Glasgow RE, Teborg JR. Worksite smoking cessation: a meta-analysis of controlled studies. *J Occup Med,* 1990, 32:429–439.

25 US Department of Health and Human Services. *Strategies to control tobacco use in the United States: a blueprint for public health action in the 1990's.* US Department of Health and Human Services, Washington, DC, National Cancer Institute, 1991 (NIH Publ. No. 92–3316).

26 COMMIT Research Group. Community Intervention Trial for Smoking Cessation (COMMIT): Summary of design and intervention. *J Natl Cancer Inst,* 1991, 83:1620–1628.

27 National Cancer Institute. *ASSIST program guidelines for tobacco-free communities.* Bethesda, MD, National Cancer Institute, 1991.

28 Luepker RV et al. Community education for cardiovascular disease prevention: Risk factor changes in the Minnesota Heart Health Program. *Am J Public Health*, 1994, 84:1383–1393.

29 Ramsay LE et al. Dietary reduction of serum cholesterol concentration: time to think again. *Br Med J*, 1991, 303:953–957.

30 Heshka S et al. Resting energy expenditure in the obese: A cross-validation and comparison of prediction equations. *J Am Diet Assoc*, 1993, 93:1031–1036.

31 Sempos C et al. Prevalence of high blood cholesterol among US adults. *J Am Med Assoc*, 1993, 269:3009–3104.

32 Mertz W et al. What are people really eating? The relation between energy intake derived from estimated diet records and intake determined to maintain body weight. *Am J Clin Nutr*, 1991, 54:291–295.

33 Black GA, Goldberg GR, Jebb SA. Critical evaluation of energy intake data using fundamental principles of energy physiology: 2. Evaluating the results of publishing surveys. *Eur J Clin Nutr*, 1991, 45:583–599.

34 Black AE et al. Measurements of total energy expenditure provide insights into the validity of dietary measurements of energy intake. *J Am Diet Assoc*, 1993, 93:572–579.

35 Prochaska JO, DiClemente CO, Norcross JC. In search of how people change: applications to addictive behaviors. *Am Psychol*, 1992, 47:1102–1114.

36 Bandura A. Self-efficacy: toward a unifying theory of behavior change. *Psychol Rev*, 1977, 94:191–215.

37 Baer JS, Holt CS, Lichtenstein E. Self-efficacy and smoking reexamined: construct validity and clinical utility. *J Consult Clin Psychol*, 1986, 54:846–852.

38 Robert Wood Johnson Foundation. *Smokeless States Initiative*. The Robert Wood Johnson Foundation, Princeton, NJ, 1993.

39 Henderson MS et al. Feasibility of a randomized trial of a low-fat diet for the prevention of breast cancer: Dietary compliance in the Women's Health Trial Vanguard Study. *Prev Med*, 1990, 19:115–133.

40 Insull W et al. Results of a randomized feasibility study of a low-fat diet. *Arch Intern Med*, 1990, 150:421–427.

41 Cohen S et al. Debunking myths about self-quitting: Evidence from 10 prospective studies of persons who attempt to quit smoking by themselves. *Am Psychol*, 1989, 44:1355–1365.

42 US Department of Health and Human Services. *The health consequences of smoking. Cardiovascular disease: a report of the Surgeon General*. US Department of Health and Human Services, Washington, DC, 1983.

43 US Department of Health and Human Services. *The health consequences of smoking. Chronic obstructive lung disease: a report of the Surgeon General*. US Department of Health and Human Services, Washington, DC, 1984.

44 Doll R, Peto R. The causes of cancer: Quantitative estimates of avoidable risks of cancer in the United States today. *J Nat Cancer Inst*, 1981, 66:1191–1309.

45 Greenwald P, Sondik E, National Cancer Institute. *Cancer control objectives for the Nation: 1985–2000*. NCI Monographs, US Department of Health and Human Services, Public Health Service, 1986.

46 Urban N et al. Analysis of the costs of a large prevention trial. *Controlled Clinical Trials*, 1990, 11:129–146.

47 Glasgow RE, McCaul KD, Fisher KJ. Participation in worksite health promotion: a critique of the literature and recommendations for future practice. *Health Educ Q*, 1993, 20:391–408.

48 White E et al. Maintenance of a low-fat diet: Follow-up of the Women's Health Trial. *Cancer Epid Biomarkers Prev*, 1992, 1:315–323.

49 Shattuck AL, White E, Kristal AR. How women's adopted low-fat diets affect their husbands. *Am J Public Health*, 1992, 82:1244–1250.

50 Martin DC et al. A comparison of bias and precision in cohort and cross-sectional designs in community intervention studies. In: *Proceedings of the Symposium on Statistical Methods for Evaluation of Intervention and Prevention Studies*, Atlanta, GA, 1990.

51 Gail MH et al. Aspects of statistical design for the Community Intervention Trial for Smoking Cessation (COMMIT). *Controlled Clin Trials*, 1992, 13:6–21.

52 Freedman LS, Green SB, Byar DP. Assessing the gain in efficiency due to matching in a community intervention study. *Stat Med*, 1990, 9:943–942.

53 Martin DC et al. The effect of matching on the power of randomized community intervention studies. *Stat Med*, 1993, 12:329–338.

54 Bracht N et al. Community ownership and program continuation following a health demonstration project. *Health Edu Res*, 1994, 9:243–255.

M. Henderson, B. Thompson and A. Kristal
Cancer Prevention Research Program,
Fred Hutchinson Cancer Research Center,
1124 Columbia, MP-702, Seattle, WA 98104, USA

Cost-effectiveness considerations in chemoprevention of cancer

J.D.F. Habbema*, A. van der Heide, J.M.H. van den Bosch and L. Bonneux

Prevention of cancer is a very attractive concept because it would reduce the burden that cancer morbidity and subsequent mortality places on our society. Chemoprevention that is directed towards cancer prevention therefore deserves our full attention. However, merely to aim at cancer prevention does not mean that this goal will necessarily be realized.

For a chemoprevention agent to have application potential, it should at least satisfy the following requirements, as is the case for other healthcare interventions:

- The agent is of proven effectiveness (effective means in this context reducing the incidence and mortality rates of the target cancer).
- Organization of the chemoprevention is feasible.
- The favourable effects of chemoprevention are not outweighed by the burden and the health risks to the population.
- The balance between effectiveness on the one hand and risks and costs on the other is acceptable.

The evidence used to assess these requirements should ideally be based on randomized trials, feasibility studies of implementing a routine chemoprevention programme, and cost-effectiveness studies or comparable evaluation research.

The aim of this paper is to present a line of reasoning which can usefully be applied in evaluating the cost-effectiveness of chemoprevention of cancer. We will not study the trial results of a real chemoprevention intervention programme. Instead, we will discuss the assumptions and results for a hypothetical situation involving the chemoprevention of female colorectal cancer by a chemopreventive agent. The intervention is to be applied to an age cohort in a particular population. We will quantify this intervention using data from the Netherlands. We will make some idealized assumptions, in order to make the interpretation of the results easier. Coverage and

*Correspondence: J.D.F. Habbema, Department of Public Health, Faculty of Medicine, Erasmus University Rotterdam, PO Box 1738, 3000 DR Rotterdam, The Netherlands.

compliance are 100%. The chemopreventive agent has a proven favourable effect, i.e. the incidence of the cancer will be reduced by a certain fraction. We will assume that this reduction begins immediately after the start of the intervention. The consequences of a time-lag will be studied later on. It is also assumed that both intervention and effectiveness last for a lifetime. The implications of some modifications to these assumptions will be discussed in later sections.

Assessing the effects and cost-effectiveness of cancer chemoprevention

The line of reasoning in the cost-effectiveness evaluation is illustrated in Fig. 1. The boxes on the left-hand side of the figure, (1), (2), (3), (4), (5), (6), (8) and (10), concern background data and assumptions, and the boxes on the right-hand side, (7), (9), (10) and (11), concern the cost-effectiveness results.

Assumptions
Life-table, box (1)
The life-table is used twice. First, it is used to determine the age-specific life expectancy (box (2)). For example, the life expectancy of females in the Netherlands, calculated from the usual cross-sectional age-specific and gender-specific mortality rates during 1980–1984 (1), is shown in Table 1. The life expectancy is equal to the average duration of a lifelong chemoprevention regimen that starts at the respective ages. (Strictly speaking, this is only true when the agent is ineffective; when the agent is effective, the number of years of treatment will increase somewhat. On the other hand, there will be some decrease when chemoprevention stops in cases where the target cancer is diagnosed.)

Incidence and survival, box (3)
The age-specific yearly incidence of female colorectal cancer in the Netherlands is given in Table 2 for four ages (2, 3). The severity of the cancer is reflected in the survival chances after diagnosis (4, 5, 6, 7). We will assume that the survival rate does not change after the introduction of a chemoprevention programme; only the incidence may change. In Table 2, we have summarized the survival curve

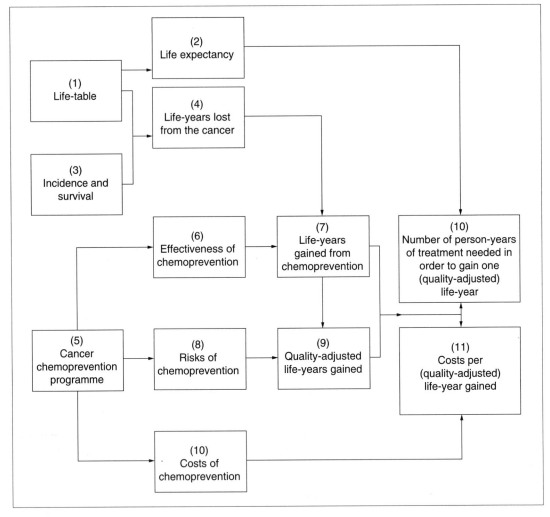

Fig. 1. Flow-chart illustrating the line of reasoning to be adopted when assessing the effects and cost-effectiveness of cancer chemoprevention.

by its expected value, i.e. the life expectancy of a female whose colorectal cancer has just been diagnosed. We prefer to use incidence and survival rather than the age-specific mortality rates from the cancer, because application of chemoprevention is linked to a reduction in incidence, and a reduction in mortality is a consequence of a lower incidence.

Loss in life expectancy, box (4)

For a female who is diagnosed as having colorectal cancer, there is a loss in life expectancy which is equal to the population life expectancy she would have experienced without the cancer minus her current incident case life expectancy. The two types of life expectancy are given in Tables 1 and 2, and the resulting loss in life expectancy is given in Table 3.

The cancer chemoprevention programme, box (5)

This programme has a target population whose life-table and cancer epidemiology have been described in boxes (1) and (3). In our example, we therefore assume that the female population in the Netherlands is offered a chemoprevention programme from a certain age onwards. We thus assume

Table 1. Life expectancy of females in the Netherlands during 1980–1984	
Age (years)	**Life expectancy (years)**
40	40.4
50	31.1
60	22.3
70	14.3

Table 2. Age-specific yearly incidence of female colorectal cancer in the Netherlands		
Age (years)	**Yearly incidence (×1000)**	**Life expectancy of an incident case (years)**
40	0.12	24.0
50	0.38	17.7
60	0.97	11.7
70	2.15	7.9

that the intervention is lifelong (it could alternatively be assumed that the chemoprevention programme only has a limited duration). For simplicity, we also assume a 100% coverage and compliance; with incomplete coverage we would have to consider the possibility of risk-selection and we would also need to specify a dose–response relationship describing how incomplete compliance affects the effectiveness of the chemoprevention.

The effectiveness of chemoprevention, box (6)

This will be expressed in terms of both the percentage reduction in the target cancer and the time-lag between the start of the chemoprevention and the time when the effects are realized. In the calculations, 10%, 25%, 50% and 100% reductions in target cancer incidence will be used. We initially assume an immediate realization of the full effect; later on, we discuss the more realistic scenario of a delay in the realization of the effects. We will not discuss the possibility that the agent has a favourable effect on other causes of death. With more complex mortality effects, the advantage of reasoning via the cancer incidence diminishes, and a direct approach via an overall mortality reduction – as, for example, observed in randomized controlled trials (RCTs) – becomes more appropriate.

The risks of chemoprevention, box (8)

These risks may vary from instantaneous and limited side-effects to (small chances of) serious morbidity, and they affect the health status of those concerned. Rather than weighing frequent small side-effects and infrequent serious risks separately, we will combine the impact of all risks into one subtraction factor to take account of a loss in the quality of life experienced by those participating in the chemoprevention programme. Quantitatively,

we assume a quality of life of 1 (on a scale of 0–1) for the women concerned in the absence of a chemoprevention programme, and an average loss in the quality of life of 1/100, 1/250 or 1/500 due to the risks of chemoprevention, resulting in quality-of-life values of 0.990, 0.996 and 0.998, respectively. In order to calculate the number of quality-adjusted life-years lived, the life-years lived have to be weighted by their quality score. For example, with a life expectancy of 40 years and a quality of life of 0.99 for the remaining years, the quality-adjusted life expectancy is 39.6 years. The risks of chemoprevention leading to mortality are not considered. If they were to exist, there would not only be a loss in quality of life, but also in life expectancy.

The costs of chemoprevention, box (10)

We will assume that the costs of the chemoprevention programme are proportional to the number

Table 3. Loss in life expectancy for a female with colorectal cancer in the Netherlands	
Age (years)	**Loss in life expectancy per cancer incidence case (years)**
40	16.4
50	13.4
60	10.6
70	6.4

Table 4. Loss in life expectancy due to colorectal cancer incidence	
Age A (years)	**Loss in life expectancy due to colorectal cancer incidence from age A onwards (years)**
40	0.376
50	0.355
60	0.307
70	0.220

of years of treatment with the agent. We thus neglect eventual fixed costs of organization, information, etc. Moreover, we will not, in this explanatory paper, consider the medical savings and costs that result from the effectiveness and the risks of chemoprevention; however, they should be included in full cost-effectiveness studies. The way in which these indirect medical costs shift the balance will differ from case to case. For example, in the context of cancer screening, we found that cervical cancer screening generates extra costs, while breast cancer screening generates some savings. Quantitatively, we will assume that the costs per year of chemoprevention treatment lie between 100 ECU and 500 ECU (on June 1, 1995, 1 ECU was equal to, for example, US$1.30, UK£0.80, FF6.50).

Results

Life-years gained by chemoprevention, box (7)

In the previous section we discussed the loss in life expectancy when colorectal cancer is diagnosed. When assessing lifelong chemoprevention, one needs to know the cumulative loss in life expectancy resulting from colorectal cancer incidence from age A (see Table 4) onwards. This quantity is calculated stepwise from older to younger ages by integrating the life-table survival, cancer incidence and subsequent loss in life expectancy. The results are given in Table 4. For example, the value for age 50 is obtained by taking the value for age 60, multiplying it by the life-table probability that someone of age 50 will reach age 60, and adding to this the additional loss between ages 50 and 60, namely the incidence between ages 50 and 60 multiplied by the associated loss in life expectancy per case. The value for

age 70 therefore uses information on older ages that has not been presented in the previous tables.

Thus, a woman aged 40 years will lose, on average, 4 months of life because of colorectal cancer; and a woman aged 70 will lose 2 months. A 100% effective chemoprevention programme will result in these amounts being added to the life expectancy. With less effective chemoprevention, i.e. when only a certain percentage of colon cancer incidence is prevented, the life-years gained will be proportionally less (see Table 5).

Quality-adjusted life-years gained, box (9)

As discussed above, we are assuming that chemoprevention has risks which lead to a decrease in the quality of life. We can now calculate the number of so-called quality-adjusted life-years gained by chemoprevention, by weighting the years lived under a chemoprevention programme with the factors 0.990, 0.996 and 0.998. Note that the two latter values correspond to a 'subtraction' of about 1 day per year lived and the value 0.990 corresponds to half a week. In this way the gain in life-years for some women as a result of chemoprevention is counteracted by a small decrease in quality of life for all. The quantitative results we obtain are given in Table 6. The rows with a quality of life of 1.0 correspond to the life-years gained in Table 5. When the quality of life is less than 1.0, the quality-adjusted life-years are obtained by subtracting an appropriate amount of the previous gain in life expectancy. For example, for an age at the start of 40 years and a quality of life of 0.998, 1/500 of the life expectancy of 40 years at age 40, i.e. 0.08 year, is subtracted from the gain in life expectancy.

Table 5. Life-years gained per woman as a result of chemoprevention of colorectal cancer			
	Effectiveness of chemoprevention		
Age at start (years)	**10%**	**25%**	**50%**	**100%**
40	0.038	0.094	0.188	0.376
50	0.036	0.089	0.178	0.355
60	0.031	0.077	0.154	0.307
70	0.022	0.055	0.110	0.220

When the loss in quality of life exceeds the original gain in life expectancy, the net value of the quality-adjusted life-years gained becomes negative; this means that chemoprevention results in a loss of quality-adjusted life-years in the target population.

The results are illuminating. They show quantitatively just how sensitive the health balance of chemoprevention is, even for small losses in health-related quality of life as a result of the risks of chemoprevention. Table 6 considers quality-of-life reductions up to 1%. When quality of life would be reduced by 1.5% (to 0.985) by chemoprevention, the balance would become negative for all starting ages of the 100% effective chemoprevention programme. Note that in these exploratory calculations, we did not make a correction for quality of life related to having colorectal cancer. This simplification probably has no serious impact on the conclusions. For cancer, by far the most pronounced loss in quality of life occurs in the very last period of life, namely the period with metastatic disease. However, mortality from other causes is also often preceded by a period of serious morbidity,

which gives rise to considerable loss in the quality of life. This will be experienced at a later age by women whose lives increase in length because of chemoprevention. We thus implicitly assumed in our calculations that the end-of-life losses in the quality of life resulting from both chemoprevention and the absence of chemoprevention cancel each other. In complete cost-effectiveness studies, this assumption, and also the assumption that the quality of life without chemoprevention has the optimal value of 1.0, should be scrutinized and possibly replaced by more realistic assumptions.

Cost-effectiveness
Number of years of chemoprevention needed
Tables 5 and 6 described the effectiveness of chemoprevention. We now turn to cost-effectiveness. An interesting and readily interpretable concept for relating resource use to effectiveness is the so-called 'number needed to treat' (NNT). The simplest NNT concept in our context would be the NNT required to prevent one incident case of colorectal cancer. We will use an NNT concept

Age at start (years)	Quality of life	Effectiveness of chemoprevention			
		10%	25%	50%	100%
40	0.990	Negative	Negative	Negative	Negative
	0.996	Negative	Negative	0.026	0.214
	0.998	Negative	0.013	0.107	0.295
	1.000	0.038	0.094	0.188	0.376
50	0.990	Negative	Negative	Negative	0.044
	0.996	Negative	Negative	0.054	0.231
	0.998	Negative	0.027	0.116	0.293
	1.000	0.036	0.089	0.178	0.355
60	0.990	Negative	Negative	Negative	0.035
	0.996	Negative	Negative	0.065	0.218
	0.998	Negative	0.032	0.109	0.262
	1.000	0.031	0.077	0.154	0.307
70	0.990	Negative	Negative	Negative	0.077
	0.996	Negative	Negative	0.053	0.163
	0.998	Negative	Negative	0.081	0.191
	1.000	0.022	0.055	0.110	0.220

Table 6. Quality-adjusted life-years gained per woman as a result of chemoprevention of colorectal cancer

Table 7. Number of years of chemopreventive treatment needed to gain 1 life-year (NYNT) in chemoprevention of female colorectal cancer

Age at start (years)	Effectiveness of chemoprevention			
	10%	25%	50%	100%
40	1074	430	215	107
50	874	350	175	87
60	726	290	145	73
70	649	260	130	65

which incorporates time (and quality of life) aspects, namely the 'number of years of chemo-preventive treatment needed in order to gain one (quality-adjusted) life-year' [NYNT; see box (10) of Fig. 1].

As discussed before, the average duration of life-long chemopreventive treatment is approximated by the life expectancy. Table 7 presents the NYNT without quality adjustment for our illustrative example of female colorectal cancer. For example, for an age at the start of a 100% effective chemo-prevention programme of 50 years, we need an average of 31.1 years of chemoprevention treatment

Table 8. Number of years of chemoprevention treatment needed (NYNT) to gain 1 quality-adjusted life-year, in a female colorectal chemoprevention programme starting at age 50

Quality of life	Effectiveness of chemoprevention			
	10%	25%	50%	100%
0.990	−113	−140	−234	707
0.996	−353	−889	576	135
0.998	−1196	1111	268	106
1.000	874	350	175	87

(namely the life expectancy at age 50) to gain 0.355 life-years (Table 5). Dividing these two numbers gives 87 years for the NYNT of this programme.

We now turn to the quality-adjusted life-years gained. Because the number of life-years gained is reduced by the quality correction, more years of treatment are needed to gain 1 life-year. This is illustrated in Table 8 for a chemoprevention pro-gramme starting at age 50. The bottom row, with-out quality correction, is identical to the '50 years' entry in Table 7. The negative values indicate how many years of treatment with a harmful chemo-preventive agent will result in the loss of 1 (quality-adjusted) life-year.

Influence of time-lag and duration of treatment

We assumed a one-step immediate total effec-tiveness of the chemoprevention. In reality there will be a gradual build-up and decline of the effec-tiveness. Of special importance for the cost-effec-tiveness is the existence of a (long) time-lag be-tween the start of chemoprevention and the influ-ence on incidence (see Table 9 for the consequences for the NYNT). With a start at a relatively young age, when cancer incidence is still low, a time-lag of 5–10 years has limited influence, but when chemoprevention starts at older ages, the impact on cost-effectiveness is considerable. On the other hand, the data on the number of years of treatment needed will become more favourable when only a limited duration of treatment is needed for a (much) longer duration of reduction in incidence. For example, when starting at age 50, lifelong treat-ment will have an average duration of 31.1 years (the life expectancy), but treatment up to age 60 will last only 8.8 years (the truncated life expectancy until age 60). Thus, with lifelong effectiveness, the NYNT figures will become a factor of 3.5 more favour-able when only treatment until age 60 is needed.

Cost-effectiveness ratio

A second measure of the relationship between resource use on the one hand and effectiveness on the other is the cost-effectiveness ratio: CER = (costs of the chemoprevention programme)/(number of quality-adjusted life-years gained by the programme).

For our illustrative calculations we assume that the costs of 1 year of treatment lie between 100 and 500 ECU (see the 'assumptions' section). Note that the CER is closely related, numerically, to the NYNT:

Table 9. Number of years of chemopreventive treatment needed to gain 1 life-year (NYNT) in chemoprevention of female colorectal cancer (assuming an immediate effect and time-lags of 5 and 10 years; we only consider the situation in which chemoprevention is 100% effective)			
	Time-lag to the start of incidence reduction (years)		
Age at start (years)	0	5	10
40	107	110	116
50	87	94	106
60	73	87	113
70	65	94	161

the denominators are identical, and the numerator of the CER is obtained by multiplying the numerator of NYNT by the costs of 1 year of treatment; thus CER = NYNT × costs of chemoprevention treatment per year.

Thus, Tables 7 and 8 can also be used for the CER, but with the appropriate factor applied. For example, when we consider a chemoprevention programme of 25% effectiveness applied to 50-year-old women, the number of years of treatment needed for a gain of 1 life-year is 350, and this figure increases to 1111 years for a gain of 1 quality-adjusted life-year when the quality of life is reduced from 1.0 to 0.998 by chemoprevention. With a cost of 100–500 ECU per year of treatment, the corresponding CER figures are 35 000–175 000 (111 000–555 000) ECU per (quality-adjusted) life-year gained. Table 10 gives the results for this case where chemoprevention is started at 50 years of

Table 10. Costs per quality-adjusted life-year gained of a female colorectal cancer chemoprevention programme which is 25% effective and starts at the age of 50		
	Cost per year of treatment	
Quality of life	100 ECU	500 ECU
0.990	−14 000	−70 000
0.996	−88 900	−444 500
0.998	111 100	555 500
1.000	35 000	175 000

age and has an effectiveness of 25%. Negative values indicate that, even though you might invest in chemoprevention, you will end up with a net loss in quality-adjusted life-years.

Discussion

Although the calculations have been confined to a hypothetical and simplified example of chemoprevention of female colorectal cancer, the methodology used is quite general. The steps in Fig. 1 can also be applied to other situations. Of course, the precision of the conclusions concerning cost-effectiveness depends crucially on the knowledge of the effects and risks of the chemoprevention. Some cost-effectiveness issues, such as discounting for time-preference, have not been discussed; Hillman et al. (8) is a recent authoritative publication of cost-effectiveness analysis. Useful textbooks include Drummond et al. (9) and Warner & Luce (10). The assessment of preventive activities is discussed in Russel (11). Colorectal cancer is one of the more common cancers. Nevertheless, from our idealized calculations it appears that effectiveness and cost-effectiveness figures could easily become unfavourable. This reinforces the point of view that chemoprevention should, in the first place, be targeted at high-risk groups.

Note that the reasoning applied in this chapter also applies to chemoprevention of metastatic disease after primary treatment, or to chemoprevention of the progression of pre-invasive lesions to invasive cancer; only the definitions of population, incidence, etc. have to be adapted to the new situation.

In a real-life chemoprevention programme there are a number of complicating factors which should be taken into account. When chemoprevention is applied to a population over a longer time period, for example, the fact that the life-table, incidence and survival may change considerably over time needs to be considered.

Compliance will, in reality, be less than 100%. This may have considerable implications for cost-effectiveness, especially when there is an association between compliance and cancer risk, in the sense that effectiveness will be reduced more than proportionally with incomplete compliance. This will be the case when women at high risk show a lower compliance with the chemoprevention programme than do women at low risk, a phenomenon that is described in cervical cancer screening. As far as effectiveness was concerned, we assumed that the chemotherapeutic agent is effective against one specific target cancer. With more complex effectiveness patterns – e.g. if several cancers are prevented with different degrees of effectiveness and perhaps other causes of death are also affected – the calculations become more complex.

In conclusion, the cost-effectiveness methodology described in the present paper provides a good framework for evaluation, but has to be adapted and refined in order to meet the characteristics of a particular chemoprevention programme.

References

1 Centraal Bureau voor de Statistiek. *Overlevingstafel naar leeftijd, 1980–1984*. The Hague, Maandstatistiek bevolking, 1986, 4:37–38.

2 Netherlands Cancer Registry. *Incidence of cancer in the Netherlands, 1989*. First report. Utrecht, Netherlands Cancer Registry, 1992.

3 Bonneux L et al. Diverging trends in colorectal cancer morbidity and mortality. Earlier diagnosis comes at a price. *Eur J Cancer*, 1995, 31:1665–1676.

4 Cancer Registry of Norway. *Survival of cancer patients. Cases diagnosed in Norway 1968–1975*. Oslo, Cancer Registry of Norway, 1980.

5 Coebergh JWW et al. Survival of cancer patients in southeastern Netherlands in the period 1975–85 (in Dutch). *Ned Tijdschr Geneeskd*, 1991, 135:935–943.

6 Enblad P et al. Improved survival of patients with cancers of the colon and rectum? *J Natl Cancer Inst*, 1988, 80:586–591.

7 Finnish Foundation for Cancer Research. *Cancer in Finland 1954–2008*, vol. 42. Helsinki, Cancer Society of Finland, 1989.

8 Task Force on Principles for Economic Analysis of Health Care Technology, Economic analysis of health care technology: A report on principles. *Ann Intern Med*, 1995, 122:61–70.

9 Drummond MF, Stoddart GL, Torrance GW. *Methods for the economic evaluation of heatlh care programmes*. New York, Oxford University Press, 1987.

10 Warner K, Luce B. *Cost-benefit and cost-effectiveness analysis in health care: principles, practice and potential*. Ann Arbor, MI, Health Administration Press, 1982.

11 Russel L. *Is prevention better than cure?* Washington, DC, The Brookings Institution, 1986.

J.D.F. Habbema, A. van der Heide, J.M.H. van den Bosch and L. Bonneux
Department of Public Health, Faculty of Medicine, Erasmus University Rotterdam, PO Box 1738, 3000 DR Rotterdam, The Netherlands

Conclusions and recommendations

V. Beral, A. Costa, R. Kroes and D.M. Parkin

1. The meeting served to update the review by E. Buiatti (IARC Technical Report No. 18) of trials in progress and those for which results had been reported. The results from two large-scale intervention studies which reported during 1994 (the ATBC prevention study in Finland and the US NCI-sponsored Linxian trial), both investigating the ability of micronutrients to reduce cancer incidence in high-risk populations, were essentially negative. (The meeting participants took a rather more sceptical view of the results from the Linxian trial than did the investigators, noting that a reduction in stomach cancer mortality was but one of multiple outcomes investigated.)

It was noted that several important trials were still in progress, which would certainly provide informative results with respect to future actions. At the same time, the existence of many small trials that would be uninformative unless results were combined in some meta-analysis was pointed out.

2. The positive results of chemoprevention to date are:

(a) in the use of tamoxifen in breast cancer patients, where there is a reduced rate of recurrence or, more meaningfully for chemoprevention, a reduced incidence of contralateral breast cancer;
(b) in the ability of retinoids (natural and synthetic) to promote regression of precancerous lesions in the oral cavity.

3. In future, evaluation might concentrate on:

(a) natural substances (rather than synthetic chemicals), which have the advantage that, if effective, they can be added to food products rather than requiring 'medication';
(b) vitamins, since these are already being widely consumed in a belief in their efficacy, and formal proof of this is required;
(c) agents that can be administered as depot preparations (to avoid problems of compliance);
(d) agents for which *a priori* evidence of effectiveness is available, either from observational studies in humans or from appropriate animal studies; in this context, it was noted that:

(i) there were few animal models available that are relevant to chemoprevention;

(ii) whenever possible, advantage should be taken of the opportunity offered by prospective studies to evaluate the effects of exposures to potential chemopreventive agents – as was done, for example, for non-steroidal anti-inflammatory drugs.

4. More care is needed in the study design of future trials.

The most important issue is to consider at what stage of the carcinogenetic process the agent is presumed to act. For example, antioxidants presumably act to reduce DNA damage at a relatively early stage, so that it was perhaps optimistic to expect them to reduce cancer incidence within periods of 5–7 years. Chemoprevention trials will generally have to be quite long (and large in size, if cancer is used as an end-point), but practical considerations of follow-up, compliance, etc. will mean that 12–15 years is really the maximum possible length. Thus, for agents that are likely to prevent early changes (e.g. to DNA), it will be necessary to study outcome in terms of intermediate end-points. These trials will generally need to be conducted early in life.

The need to conduct more work on validating the predictive value of intermediate end-points for cancer outcomes was stressed. The end-points must be distinguished from markers of exposure. In future, relatively specific changes in DNA that are predictive of particular cancers will probably be available.

5. High-risk groups are particularly appropriate for trials, primarily from a logistical viewpoint (they can be much smaller), before proceeding (if appropriate) to extrapolations or to actual interventions within the general population. High-risk groups might be:

(a) cancer patients who are known to be at high risk of a second primary cancer;
(b) individuals recognized as having specific genetic predispositions, either inherited (e.g. BRCA1) or acquired through presumed earlier environmental exposures;
(c) population subgroups with known behaviours or exposures putting them at high risk [e.g. asbestos-exposed (lung), sun-exposed (skin), hepatitis virus carriers (liver)].

6. The potential toxicity of chemopreventive agents is an important issue from the ethical viewpoint (although it was noted that many chemopreventive agents – e.g. vitamins – are only subject to warnings about toxicity if they are given as part of a trial, and not when self-acquired).

Toxicity is often evaluated concurrently with trials of preventive efficacy, as in the case of tamoxifen.

7. Cost-effectiveness of chemoprevention is clearly important from a public health viewpoint, and has important implications for the implementation of the programmes. Trials exist to quantify effectiveness (if any) and provide the data upon which such evaluations can be based.

8. Ethical considerations relate in part to the balance of risks and benefits. Small risks, both medical (e.g. toxicity) and psycho-social, run by large numbers of otherwise healthy individuals may add up to a larger negative outcome than the benefits, which for any given individual have a low probability, are unpredictable and occur late.

9. Behavioural intervention was considered as an alternative to chemoprevention. Normally, it is applicable to entire populations and results in modest changes to the average population-level risk. Behavioural interventions do, however, have certain other advantages over chemoprevention, which make them interesting from a public health viewpoint: additional benefits may accrue to future generations, there should be few side-effects, and the biological basis for effectiveness does not necessarily require to be understood (e.g. for dietary changes such as increased fruit and vegetable consumption). Nevertheless, from an individual's viewpoint, chemoprevention may be less difficult to adopt than lifestyle changes, as witnessed by vitamin consumption in the United States.

V. Beral
ICRF Cancer Epidemiology Unit, University of Oxford, Oxford OX2 6HE, United Kingdom

A. Costa
European Institute of Oncology, Via Ripamonti 435, 20141 Milan, Italy

R. Kroes
Rijksinstituut voor Volksgezondheid en Millieuhygiene, Antonie van Leeuwenhoeklaan 9, NL-3720 BA Bilthoven, The Netherlands

D.M. Parkin
Unit of Descriptive Epidemiology, International Agency for Research on Cancer, 150 cours Albert Thomas, 69372 Lyon cedex 08, France

IARC Monographs on the Evaluation of Carcinogenic Risks to Humans

Volume 1
Some Inorganic Substances, Chlorinated Hydrocarbons, Aromatic Amines, N-Nitroso Compounds, and Natural Products
1972; 184 pages; ISBN 92 832 1201 0
(out of print)

Volume 2
Some Inorganic and Organometallic Compounds
1973; 181 pages; ISBN 92 832 1202 9
(out of print)

Volume 3
Certain Polycyclic Aromatic Hydrocarbons and Heterocyclic Compounds
1973; 271 pages; ISBN 92 832 1203 7
(out of print)

Volume 4
Some Aromatic Amines, Hydrazine and Related Substances, N-Nitroso Compounds and Miscellaneous Alkylating Agents
1974; 286 pages; ISBN 92 832 1204 5
Sw. fr. 24

Volume 5
Some Organochlorine Pesticides
1974; 241 pages; ISBN 92 832 1205 3
(out of print)

Volume 6
Sex Hormones
1974; 243 pages; ISBN 92 832 1206 1
(out of print)

Volume 7
Some Anti-Thyroid and Related Substances, Nitrofurans and Industrial Chemicals
1974; 326 pages; ISBN 92 832 1207 X
(out of print)

Volume 8
Some Aromatic Azo Compounds
1975; 357 pages; ISBN 92 832 1208 8
Sw. fr. 44

Volume 9
Some Aziridines, N-, S- and O-Mustards and Selenium
1975; 268 pages; ISBN 92 832 1209 6
Sw. fr. 33

Volume 10
Some Naturally Occurring Substances
1976; 353 pages; ISBN 92 832 1210 X
(out of print)

Volume 11
Cadmium, Nickel, Some Epoxides, Miscellaneous Industrial Chemicals and General Considerations on Volatile Anaesthetics
1976; 306 pages; ISBN 92 832 1211 8
(out of print)

Volume 12
Some Carbamates, Thiocarbamates and Carbazides
1976; 282 pages; ISBN 92 832 1212 6
Sw. fr. 41

Volume 13
Some Miscellaneous Pharmaceutical Substances
1977; 255 pages; ISBN 92 832 1213 4
Sw. fr. 36

Volume 14
Asbestos
1977; 106 pages; ISBN 92 832 1214 2
(out of print)

Volume 15
Some Fumigants, the Herbicides 2,4-D and 2,4,5-T, Chlorinated Dibenzodioxins and Miscellaneous Industrial Chemicals
1977; 354 pages; ISBN 92 832 1215 0
(out of print)

Volume 16
Some Aromatic Amines and Related Nitro Compounds – Hair Dyes, Colouring Agents and Miscellaneous Industrial Chemicals
1978; 400 pages; ISBN 92 832 1216 9
Sw. fr. 60

Volume 17
Some N-Nitroso Compounds
1978; 365 pages; ISBN 92 832 1217 7
Sw. fr. 60

Volume 18
Polychlorinated Biphenyls and Polybrominated Biphenyls
1978; 140 pages; ISBN 92 832 1218 5
Sw. fr. 24

Volume 19
Some Monomers, Plastics and Synthetic Elastomers, and Acrolein
1979; 513 pages; ISBN 92 832 1219 3
(out of print)

Volume 20
Some Halogenated Hydrocarbons
1979; 609 pages; ISBN 92 832 1220 7
(out of print)

Volume 21
Sex Hormones (II)
1979; 583 pages; ISBN 92 832 1521 4
Sw. fr. 72

Volume 22
Some Non-Nutritive Sweetening Agents
1980; 208 pages; ISBN 92 832 1522 2
Sw. fr. 30

Volume 23
Some Metals and Metallic Compounds
1980; 438 pages; ISBN 92 832 1523 0
(out of print)

Volume 24
Some Pharmaceutical Drugs
1980; 337 pages; ISBN 92 832 1524 9
Sw. fr. 48

Volume 25
Wood, Leather and Some Associated Industries
1981; 412 pages; ISBN 92 832 1525 7
Sw. fr. 72

Volume 26
Some Antineoplastic and Immunosuppressive Agents
1981; 411 pages; ISBN 92 832 1526 5
Sw. fr. 75

Volume 27
Some Aromatic Amines, Anthraquinones and Nitroso Compounds, and Inorganic Fluorides Used in Drinking Water and Dental Preparations
1982; 341 pages; ISBN 92 832 1527 3
Sw. fr. 48

Volume 28
The Rubber Industry
1982; 486 pages; ISBN 92 832 1528 1
Sw. fr. 84

Volume 29
Some Industrial Chemicals and Dyestuffs
1982; 416 pages; ISBN 92 832 1529 X
Sw. fr. 72

Volume 30
Miscellaneous Pesticides
1983; 424 pages; ISBN 92 832 1530 3
Sw. fr. 72

Volume 31
Some Food Additives, Feed Additives and Naturally Occurring Substances
1983; 314 pages; ISBN 92 832 1531 1
Sw. fr. 66

IARC Scientific Publications

No. 16
Air Pollution and Cancer in Man
Edited by U. Mohr, D. Schmähl and
L. Tomatis
1977; 328 pages; ISBN 0 19 723015 6
US$ 20

No. 17
**Directory of On-Going Research in
Cancer Epidemiology 1977**
Edited by C.S. Muir and G. Wagner
1977; 599 pages; ISBN 92 832 1117 0
(out of print)

No. 18
**Environmental Carcinogens. Selected
Methods of Analysis. Volume 1:
Analysis of Volatile Nitrosamines in
Food**
Editor-in-Chief: H. Egan
1978; 212 pages; ISBN 0 19 723017 2
US$ 15

No. 19
**Environmental Aspects of
N-Nitroso Compounds**
Edited by E.A. Walker, M. Castegnaro,
L. Griciute and R.E. Lyle
1978; 561 pages; ISBN 0 19 723018 0
US$ 30

No. 20
**Nasopharyngeal Carcinoma: Etiology
and Control**
Edited by G. de Thé and Y. Ito
1978; 606 pages; ISBN 0 19 723019 9
US$ 30

No. 21
**Cancer Registration and its
Techniques**
Edited by R. MacLennan, C. Muir,
R. Steinitz and A. Winkler
1978; 235 pages; ISBN 0 19 723020 2
US$ 20

No. 22
**Environmental Carcinogens:
Selected Methods of Analysis.
Volume 2: Methods for the
Measurement of Vinyl Chloride in
Poly(vinyl chloride), Air, Water and
Foodstuffs**
Editor-in-Chief: H. Egan
1978; 142 pages; ISBN 0 19 723021 0
US$ 15

No. 23
**Pathology of Tumours in Laboratory
Animals.
Volume II: Tumours of
the Mouse**
Editor-in-Chief: V.S. Turusov
1979; 669 pages; ISBN 0 19 723022 9
US$ 20

No. 24
Oncogenesis and Herpesviruses III
Edited by G. de-Thé, W. Henle and
F. Rapp
1978; Part I: 580 pages, Part II: 512
pages; ISBN 0 19 723023 7
US$ 40

No. 25
**Carcinogenic Risk: Strategies for
Intervention**
Edited by W. Davis and C. Rosenfeld
1979; 280 pages; ISBN 0 19 723025 3
US$ 20

No. 26
**Directory of On-going Research in
Cancer Epidemiology 1978**
Edited by C.S. Muir and G. Wagner
1978; 550 pages; ISBN 0 19 723026 1
(out of print)

No. 27
**Molecular and Cellular Aspects of
Carcinogen Screening Tests**
Edited by R. Montesano, H. Bartsch and
L. Tomatis
1980; 372 pages; ISBN 0 19 723027 X
£30.00, US$ 20

No. 28
**Directory of On-going Research in
Cancer Epidemiology 1979**
Edited by C.S. Muir and G. Wagner
1979; 672 pages; ISBN 92 832 1128 6
(out of print)

No. 29
**Environmental Carcinogens.
Selected Methods of Analysis.
Volume 3: Analysis of Polycyclic
Aromatic Hydrocarbons in
Environmental Samples**
Editor-in-Chief: H. Egan
1979; 240 pages; ISBN 0 19 723028 8
US$ 15

No. 30
Biological Effects of Mineral Fibres
Editor-in-Chief: J.C. Wagner
1980; Two volumes, 494 pages &
513 pages; ISBN 0 19 723030 X
US$ 40

No. 31
**N-Nitroso Compounds: Analysis,
Formation and Occurrence**
Edited by E.A. Walker, L. Griciute,
M. Castegnaro and M. Börzsönyi
1980; 835 pages; ISBN 0 19 723031 8
US$ 30

No. 32
**Statistical Methods in Cancer
Research. Volume 1: The Analysis of**

Case-control Studies
By N.E. Breslow and N.E. Day
1980; 338 pages; ISBN 92 832 0132 9
£ 18

No. 33
**Handling Chemical Carcinogens in
the Laboratory**
Edited by R. Montesano, H. Bartsch,
E. Boyland, G. Della Porta, L. Fishbein,
R.A. Griesemer, A.B. Swan and
L. Tomatis
1979; 32 pages; ISBN 0 19 723033 4
(out of print)

No. 34
**Pathology of Tumours in
Laboratory Animals.
Volume III: Tumours of the
Hamster**
Editor-in-Chief: V.S. Turusov
1982; 461 pages; ISBN 0 19 723034 2
US$ 30

No. 35
**Directory of On-going Research in
Cancer Epidemiology 1980**
Edited by C.S. Muir and G. Wagner
1980; 660 pages; ISBN 0 19 723035 0
(out of print)

No. 36
**Cancer Mortality by Occupation and
Social Class 1851–1971**
Edited by W.P.D. Logan
1982; 253 pages; ISBN 0 19 723036 9
US$ 20

No. 37
**Laboratory Decontamination
and Destruction of Aflatoxins
B1, B2, G1, G2 in Laboratory
Wastes**
Edited by M. Castegnaro,
D.C. Hunt, E.B. Sansone,
P.L. Schuller, M.G. Siriwardana,
G.M. Telling, H.P. van Egmond and
E.A. Walker
1980; 56 pages; ISBN 0 19 723037 7
US$ 8

No. 38
**Directory of On-going Research in
Cancer Epidemiology 1981**
Edited by C.S. Muir and G. Wagner
1981; 696 pages; ISBN 0 19 723038 5
(out of print)

No. 39
**Host Factors in Human
Carcinogenesis**
Edited by H. Bartsch and B. Armstrong
1982; 583 pages;
ISBN 0 19 723039 3
US$ 30

No. 62
Directory of On-going Research in Cancer Epidemiology 1984
Edited by C.S. Muir and G. Wagner
1984; 717 pages; ISBN 0 19 723062 8
(out of print)

No. 63
Virus-associated Cancers in Africa
Edited by A.O. Williams, G.T. O'Conor, G.B. de Thé and C.A. Johnson
1984; 773 pages; ISBN 0 19 723063 6
US$ 30

No. 64
Laboratory Decontamination and Destruction of Carcinogens in Laboratory Wastes: Some Aromatic Amines and 4-Nitrobiphenyl
Edited by M. Castegnaro, J. Barek, J. Dennis, G. Ellen, M. Klibanov, M. Lafontaine, R. Mitchum, P. van Roosmalen, E.B. Sansone, L.A. Sternson and M. Vahl
1985; 84 pages; ISBN: 92 832 1164 2
US$ 8

No. 65
Interpretation of Negative Epidemiological Evidence for Carcinogenicity
Edited by N.J. Wald and R. Doll
1985; 232 pages; ISBN 92 832 1165 0
US$ 15

No. 66
The Role of the Registry in Cancer Control
Edited by D.M. Parkin, G. Wagner and C.S. Muir
1985; 152 pages; ISBN 92 832 0166 3
£ 10

No. 67
Transformation Assay of Established Cell Lines: Mechanisms and Application
Edited by T. Kakunaga and H. Yamasaki
1985; 225 pages; ISBN 92 832 1167 7
US$ 15

No. 68
Environmental Carcinogens: Selected Methods of Analysis. Volume 7: Some Volatile Halogenated Hydrocarbons
Edited by L. Fishbein and I.K. O'Neill
1985; 479 pages; ISBN 92 832 1168 5
US$ 30

No. 69
Directory of On-going Research in Cancer Epidemiology 1985
Edited by C.S. Muir and G. Wagner
1985; 745 pages; ISBN 92 823 1169 3
(out of print)

No. 70
The Role of Cyclic Nucleic Acid Adducts in Carcinogenesis and Mutagenesis
Edited by B. Singer and H. Bartsch
1986; 467 pages; ISBN 92 832 1170 7
US$ 30

No. 71
Environmental Carcinogens: Selected Methods of Analysis. Volume 8: Some Metals: As, Be, Cd, Cr, Ni, Pb, Se, Zn
Edited by I.K. O'Neill, P. Schuller and L. Fishbein
1986; 485 pages; ISBN 92 832 1171 5
US$ 30

No. 72
Atlas of Cancer in Scotland, 1975–1980: Incidence and Epidemiological Perspective
Edited by I. Kemp, P. Boyle, M. Smans and C.S. Muir
1985; 285 pages; ISBN 92 832 1172 3
US$ 20

No. 73
Laboratory Decontamination and Destruction of Carcinogens in Laboratory Wastes: Some Antineoplastic Agents
Edited by M. Castegnaro, J. Adams, M.A. Armour, J. Barek, J. Benvenuto, C. Confalonieri, U. Goff, G. Telling
1985; 163 pages; ISBN 92 832 1173 1
£ 13.50

No. 74
Tobacco: A Major International Health Hazard
Edited by D. Zaridze and R. Peto
1986; 324 pages; ISBN 92 832 1174 X
£ 24

No. 75
Cancer Occurrence in Developing Countries
Edited by D.M. Parkin
1986; 339 pages; ISBN 92 832 1175 8
£ 24

No. 76
Screening for Cancer of the Uterine Cervix
Edited by M. Hakama, A.B. Miller and N.E. Day
1986; 315 pages; ISBN 92 832 1176 6
£ 31.50

No. 77
Hexachlorobenzene: Proceedings of an International Symposium
Edited by C.R. Morris and J.R.P. Cabral
1986; 668 pages; ISBN 92 832 1177 4
US$ 40

No. 78
Carcinogenicity of Alkylating Cytostatic Drugs
Edited by D. Schmähl and J.M. Kaldor
1986; 337 pages; ISBN 92 832 1178 2
US$ 20

No. 79
Statistical Methods in Cancer Research. Volume III: The Design and Analysis of Long-term Animal Experiments
By J.J. Gart, D. Krewski, P.N. Lee, R.E. Tarone and J. Wahrendorf
1986; 213 pages; ISBN 92 832 1179 0
£ 23.50

No. 80
Directory of On-going Research in Cancer Epidemiology 1986
Edited by C.S. Muir and G. Wagner
1986; 805 pages; ISBN 92 832 1180 4
(out of print)

No. 81
Environmental Carcinogens: Methods of Analysis and Exposure Measurement. Volume 9: Passive Smoking
Edited by I.K. O'Neill, K.D. Brunnemann, B. Dodet and D. Hoffmann
1987; 383 pages; ISBN 92 832 1181 2
£ 37

No. 82
Statistical Methods in Cancer Research. Volume II: The Design and Analysis of Cohort Studies
By N.E. Breslow and N.E. Day
1987; 404 pages; ISBN 92 832 0182 5
£ 25

No. 83
Long-term and Short-term Assays for Carcinogens: A Critical Appraisal
Edited by R. Montesano, H. Bartsch, H. Vainio, J. Wilbourn and H. Yamasaki
1986; 575 pages; ISBN 92 832 1183 9
£ 37

No. 84
The Relevance of N-Nitroso Compounds to Human Cancer: Exposure and Mechanisms
Edited by H. Bartsch, I.K. O'Neill and R. Schulte-Hermann
1987; 671 pages; ISBN 92 832 1184 7
US$ 40

No. 85
Environmental Carcinogens: Methods of Analysis and Exposure Measurement. Volume 10: Benzene and Alkylated Benzenes
Edited by L. Fishbein and I.K. O'Neill
1988; 327 pages; ISBN 92 832 1185 5
£42

No. 86
Directory of On-going Research in Cancer Epidemiology 1987
Edited by D.M. Parkin and
J. Wahrendorf
1987; 685 pages; ISBN: 92 832 1186 3
(out of print)

No. 87
International Incidence of Childhood Cancer
Edited by D.M. Parkin, C.A. Stiller,
C.A. Bieber, G.J. Draper. B. Terracini
and J.L. Young
1988; 401 page; ISBN 92 832 1187 1
(out of print)

No. 88
Cancer Incidence in Five Continents, Volume V
Edited by C. Muir, J. Waterhouse,
T. Mack, J. Powell and S. Whelan
1987; 1004 pages; ISBN 92 832 1188 X
£ 58

No. 89
Methods for Detecting DNA Damaging Agents in Humans: Applications in Cancer Epidemiology and Prevention
Edited by H. Bartsch, K. Hemminki and
I.K. O'Neill
1988; 518 pages; ISBN 92 832 1189 8
(out of print)

No. 90
Non-occupational Exposure to Mineral Fibres
Edited by J. Bignon, J. Peto and
R. Saracci
1989; 500 pages; ISBN 92 832 1190 1
£ 52.50

No. 91
Trends in Cancer Incidence in Singapore 1968–1982
Edited by H.P. Lee, N.E. Day and
K. Shanmugaratnam
1988; 160 pages; ISBN 92 832 1191 X
US$ 20

No. 92
Cell Differentiation, Genes and Cancer
Edited by T. Kakunaga, T. Sugimura,
L. Tomatis and H. Yamasaki
1988; 204 pages; ISBN 92 832 1192 8
£ 29

No. 93
Directory of On-going Research in Cancer Epidemiology 1988
Edited by M. Coleman and J. Wahrendorf
1988; 662 pages; ISBN 92 832 1193 6
(out of print)

No. 94
Human Papillomavirus and Cervical Cancer
Edited by N. Muñoz, F.X. Bosch and
O.M. Jensen
1989; 154 pages; ISBN 92 832 1194 4
£ 22.50

No. 95
Cancer Registration: Principles and Methods
Edited by O.M. Jensen, D.M. Parkin, R. MacLennan, C.S. Muir and R. Skeet
1991; 296 pages; ISBN 92 832 1195 2
£ 28

No. 96
Perinatal and Multigeneration Carcinogenesis
Edited by N.P. Napalkov, J.M. Rice,
L. Tomatis and H. Yamasaki
1989; 436 pages; ISBN 92 832 1196 0
£ 52.50

No. 97
Occupational Exposure to Silica and Cancer Risk
Edited by L. Simonato, A.C. Fletcher,
R. Saracci and T. Thomas
1990; 124 pages; ISBN 92 832 1197 9
£ 24

No. 98
Cancer Incidence in Jewish Migrants to Israel, 1961-1981
Edited by R. Steinitz, D.M. Parkin,
J.L. Young, C.A. Bieber and L. Katz
1989; 320 pages; ISBN 92 832 1198 7
£ 37

No. 99
Pathology of Tumours in Laboratory Animals, Second Edition, Volume 1, Tumours of the Rat
Edited by V.S. Turusov and U. Mohr
1990; 740 pages; ISBN 92 832 1199 5
£ 90
For Volumes 2 and 3 (Tumours of the Mouse and Tumours of the Hamster), see IARC Scientific Publications Nos. 111 and 126.

No. 100
Cancer: Causes, Occurrence and Control
Editor-in-Chief: L. Tomatis
1990; 352 pages; ISBN 92 832 0110 8
£ 25.50

No. 101
Directory of On-going Research in Cancer Epidemiology 1989–1990
Edited by M. Coleman and J. Wahrendorf
1989; 828 pages; ISBN 92 832 2101 X
£ 42

No. 102
Patterns of Cancer in Five Continents
Edited by S.L. Whelan, D.M. Parkin and
E. Masuyer
1990; 160 pages; ISBN 92 832 2102 8
£ 26.50

No. 103
Evaluating Effectiveness of Primary Prevention of Cancer
Edited by M. Hakama, V. Beral,
J.W. Cullen and D.M. Parkin
1990; 206 pages; ISBN 92 832 2103 6
£ 34

No. 104
Complex Mixtures and Cancer Risk
Edited by H. Vainio, M. Sorsa and
A.J. McMichael
1990; 441 pages; ISBN 92 832 2104 4
£ 40

No. 105
Relevance to Human Cancer of N-Nitroso Compounds, Tobacco Smoke and Mycotoxins
Edited by I.K. O'Neill, J. Chen and
H. Bartsch
1991; 614 pages; ISBN 92 832 2105 2
£ 74

No. 106
Atlas of Cancer Incidence in the Former German Democratic Republic
Edited by W.H. Mehnert, M. Smans,
C.S. Muir, M. Möhner and D. Schön
1992; 384 pages; ISBN 92 832 2106 0
£ 52.50

No. 107
Atlas of Cancer Mortality in the European Economic Community
Edited by M. Smans, C. Muir and
P. Boyle
1992; 213 pages +44 coloured maps;
ISBN 92 832 2107 9
£ 35

No. 108
Environmental Carcinogens: Methods of Analysis and Exposure Measurement. Volume 11: Polychlorinated Dioxins and Dibenzofurans
Edited by C. Rappe, H.R. Buser,
B. Dodet and I.K. O'Neill
1991; 400 pages; ISBN 92 832 2108 7
£ 47.50

No. 109
Environmental Carcinogens: Methods of Analysis and Exposure Measurement. Volume 12: Indoor Air
Edited by B. Seifert, H. van de Wiel,
B. Dodet and I.K. O'Neill
1993; 385 pages; ISBN 92 832 2109 5
£ 45

No. 110
Directory of On-going Research in Cancer Epidemiology 1991
Edited by M.P. Coleman and
J. Wahrendorf
1991; 753 pages; ISBN 92 832 2110 9
£ 40

No. 111
Pathology of Tumours in Laboratory Animals, Second Edition. Volume 2: Tumours of the Mouse
Edited by V. Turusov and U. Mohr
1994; 800 pages; ISBN 92 832 2111 1
£ 90

No. 112
Autopsy in Epidemiology and Medical Research
Edited by E. Riboli and M. Delendi
1991; 288 pages; ISBN 92 832 2112 5
£ 26.50

No. 113
Laboratory Decontamination and Destruction of Carcinogens in Laboratory Wastes: Some Mycotoxins
Edited by M. Castegnaro, J. Barek,
J.M. Frémy, M. Lafontaine, M. Miraglia,
E.B. Sansone and G.M. Telling
1991; 63 pages; ISBN 92 832 2113 3
£ 12

No. 114
Laboratory Decontamination and Destruction of Carcinogens in Laboratory Wastes: Some Polycyclic Heterocyclic Hydrocarbons
Edited by M. Castegnaro, J. Barek,
J. Jacob, U. Kirso, M. Lafontaine,
E.B. Sansone, G.M. Telling and
T. Vu Duc
1991; 50 pages; ISBN 92 832 2114 1
£ 8

No. 115
Mycotoxins, Endemic Nephropathy and Urinary Tract Tumours
Edited by M. Castegnaro, R. Plestina,
G. Dirheimer, I.N. Chernozemsky and
H. Bartsch
1991; 340 pages; ISBN 92 832 2115 X
£ 47

No. 116
Mechanisms of Carcinogenesis in Risk Identification
Edited by H. Vainio, P. Magee,
D. McGregor and A.J. McMichael
1992; 615 pages;
ISBN 92 832 2116 8
£ 69

No. 117
Directory of On-going Research in Cancer Epidemiology 1992
Edited by M. Coleman, E. Demaret and
J. Wahrendorf
1992; 773 pages;
ISBN 92 832 2117 6
£ 44.50

No. 118
Cadmium in the Human Environment: Toxicity and Carcinogenicity
Edited by G.F. Nordberg, R.F.M. Herber
and L. Alessio
1992; 470 pages;
ISBN 92 832 2118 4
£ 60

No. 119
The Epidemiology of Cervical Cancer and Human Papillomavirus
Edited by N. Muñoz, F.X. Bosch,
K.V. Shah and A. Meheus
1992; 288 pages;
ISBN 92 832 2119 2
£ 29.50

No. 120
Cancer Incidence in Five Continents, Vol. VI
Edited by D.M. Parkin, C.S. Muir,
S.L. Whelan, Y.T. Gao, J. Ferlay and
J. Powell
1992; 1020 pages;
ISBN 92 832 2120 6
£ 120

No. 121
Time Trends in Cancer Incidence and Mortality
By M. Coleman, J. Estéve, P. Damiecki,
A. Arslan and H. Renard
1993; 820 pages;
ISBN 92 832 2121 4
£ 120

No. 122
International Classification of Rodent Tumours.
Part I. The Rat
Editor-in-Chief: U. Mohr
1992–1996; 10 fascicles of 60–100
pages; ISBN 92 832 2122 2
£ 15 each

No. 123
Cancer in Italian Migrant Populations
Edited by M. Geddes, D.M. Parkin,
M. Khlat, D. Balzi and E. Buiatti
1993; 292 pages;
ISBN 92 832 2123 0
£ 40

No. 124
Postlabelling Methods for the Detection of DNA Damage
Edited by D.H. Phillips,
M. Castegnaro and H. Bartsch
1993; 392 pages;
ISBN 92 832 2124 9
£ 46

No. 125
DNA Adducts: Identification and Biological Significance
Edited by K. Hemminki, A. Dipple,
D.E.G. Shuker, F.F. Kadlubar,
D. Segerbäck and H. Bartsch
1994; 478 pages; ISBN 92 832 2125 7
£ 52

No. 128
Statistical Methods in Cancer Research. Volume IV. Descriptive Epidemiology
By J. Estève, E. Benhamou and
L. Raymond
1994; 302 pages;
ISBN 92 832 2128 1
£ 25

No. 129
Occupational Cancer in Developing Countries
Edited by N. Pearce, E. Matos,
H. Vainio, P. Boffetta and M. Kogevinas
1994; 191 pages;
ISBN 92 832 2129 X
£ 20

No. 130
Directory of On-going Research in Cancer Epidemiology 1994
Edited by R. Sankaranarayanan,
J. Wahrendorf and E. Démaret
1994; 800 pages;
ISBN 92 832 2130 3
£ 52

No. 132
Survival of Cancer Patients in Europe: The EUROCARE Study
Edited by F. Berrino, M. Sant,
A. Verdecchia, R. Capocaccia,
T. Hakulinen and J. Estève
1995; 463 pages;
ISBN 92 832 2132 X
£ 45

No. 134
Atlas of Cancer Mortality in Central Europe
W. Zatonski, J. Estéve, M. Smans,
J. Tyczynski and P. Boyle
1996 300 pages;
ISBN 92 832 2134 6
£ 45

IARC Technical Reports

No. 1
Cancer in Costa Rica
Edited by R. Sierra, R. Barrantes,
G. Muñoz Leiva, D.M. Parkin,
C.A. Bieber and N. Muñoz Calero
1988; 124 pages; ISBN 92 832 1412 9
Sw. fr. 30

No. 2
SEARCH: A Computer Package to
Assist the Statistical Analysis of
Case-Control Studies
Edited by G.J. Macfarlane, P. Boyle and
P. Maisonneuve
1991; 80 pages; ISBN 92 832 1413 7
(out of print)

No. 3
Cancer Registration in the European
Economic Community
Edited by M.P. Coleman and E. Démaret
1988; 188 pages; ISBN 92 832 1414 5
Sw. fr. 30

No. 4
Diet, Hormones and Cancer:
Methodological Issues for
Prospective Studies
Edited by E. Riboli and R. Saracci
1988; 156 pages; ISBN 92 832 1415 3
Sw. fr. 30

No. 5
Cancer in the Philippines
Edited by A.V. Laudico, D. Esteban and
D.M. Parkin
1989; 186 pages; ISBN 92 832 1416 1
Sw. fr. 30

No. 6
La genèse du Centre international de
recherche sur le cancer
By R. Sohier and A.G.B. Sutherland
1990; 102 pages; ISBN 92 832 1418 8
Sw. fr. 30

No. 7
Epidémiologie du cancer dans les
pays de langue latine
1990, 292 pages; ISBN 92 832 1419 6
Sw. fr. 30

No. 8
Comparative Study of Anti-smoking
Legislation in Countries of the
European Economic Community
By A. J. Sasco, P. Dalla-Vorgia and
P. Van der Elst
1992; 82 pages; ISBN: 92 832 1421 8
Sw. fr. 30

No. 8
(French translation) TR8F
Etude comparative des Législations

de Contrôle du Tabagisme dans les
Pays de la Communauté économique
européenne
1995; 82 pages; ISBN 92 832 2402 7
Sw. fr. 30

No. 9
Epidémiologie du cancer dans les
pays de langue latine
1991; 346 pages; ISBN 92 832 1423 4
Sw. fr. 30

No. 10
Manual for Cancer Registry
Personnel
Edited by D. Esteban, S. Whelan,
A. Laudico and D.M. Parkin
1995; 400 pages; ISBN 92 832 1424 2
Sw. fr. 45

No. 11
Nitroso Compounds: Biological
Mechanisms, Exposures and Cancer
Etiology
Edited by I. O'Neill and H. Bartsch
1992; 150 pages; ISBN 92 832 1425 X
Sw. fr. 30

No. 12
Epidémiologie du cancer dans les
pays de langue latine
1992; 375 pages; ISBN 92 832 1426 9
Sw. fr. 30

No. 13
Health, Solar UV Radiation and
Environmental Change
By A. Kricker, B.K. Armstrong,
M.E. Jones and R.C. Burton
1993; 213 pages; ISBN 92 832 1427 7
Sw. fr. 30

No. 14
Epidémiologie du cancer dans les
pays de langue latine
1993; 400 pages; ISBN 92 832 1428 5
Sw. fr. 30

No. 15
Cancer in the African Population of
Bulawayo, Zimbabwe, 1963–1977
By M.E.G. Skinner, D.M. Parkin,
A.P. Vizcaino and A. Ndhlovu
1993; 120 pages; ISBN 92 832 1429 3
Sw. fr. 30

No. 16
Cancer in Thailand 1984–1991
By V. Vatanasapt, N. Martin,
H. Sriplung, K. Chindavijak,
S. Sontipong, S. Sriamporn, D.M. Parkin
and J. Ferlay
1993; 164 pages; ISBN 92 832 1430 7
Sw. fr. 30

No. 18
Intervention Trials for Cancer
Prevention
By E. Buiatti
1994; 52 pages; ISBN 92 832 1432 3
Sw. fr. 30

No. 19
Comparability and Quality Control in
Cancer Registration
By D.M. Parkin, V.W. Chen, J. Ferlay,
J. Galceran, H.H. Storm and
S.L. Whelan
1994; 110 pages plus diskette;
ISBN 92 832 1433 1
Sw. fr. 30

No. 20
Epidémiologie du cancer dans les
pays de langue latine
1994; 346 pages; ISBN 92 832 1434 X
Sw. fr. 30

No. 21
ICD Conversion Programs for Cancer
By J. Ferlay
1994; 24 pages plus diskette;
ISBN 92 832 1435 8
Sw. fr. 30

No. 22
Cancer in Tianjin
By Q.S. Wang, P. Boffetta,
M. Kogevinas and D.M. Parkin
1994; 96 pages; ISBN 92 832 1433 1
Sw. fr. 30

No. 23
An Evaluation Programme for Cancer
Preventive Agents
By Bernard W. Stewart
1995; 40 pages; ISBN 92 832 1438 2
Sw. fr. 20

No. 24
Peroxisome Proliferation and its Role
in Carcinogenesis
1995; 85 pages;
ISBN 92 832 1439 0
Sw. fr. 30

No. 25
Combined Analysis of Cancer
Mortality in Nuclear Workers in
Canada, the United Kingdom and the
United States of America
By E. Cardis, E.S. Gilbert, L. Carpenter,
G. Howe, I. Kato, J. Fix, L. Salmon,
G. Cowper, B.K. Armstrong, V. Beral,
A. Douglas, S.A. Fry, J. Kaldor, C. Lavé,
P.G. Smith, G. Voelz and L. Wiggs
1995; 160 pages;
ISBN 92 832 1440 4
Sw. fr. 30

Directories of Agents being Tested for Carcinogenicity
Edited by M.-J. Ghess, J.D. Wilbourn and H. Vainio

No. 14
1990; 369 pages;
ISBN 92 832 1314 9
Sw. fr. 45

No. 15
1992; 317 pages; ISBN 92 832 1315 7
Sw. fr. 60

No. 16
1994; 294 pages; ISBN 92 832 1316 5
Sw. fr. 50

Non-serial publications
Alcool et Cancer
By A. Tuyns
1978; 48 pages
Fr. fr. 35

Cancer Morbidity and Causes of Death among Danish Brewery Workers
By O.M. Jensen
1980; 143 pages
Fr. fr. 75

Directory of Computer Systems Used in Cancer Registries
By H.R. Menck and D.M. Parkin
1986; 236 pages
Fr. fr. 50

Facts and Figures of Cancer in the European Community
By J. Estève, A. Kricker, J. Ferlay and D.M. Parkin
1993; 52 pages;
ISBN 92 832 1437 4
Sw. fr. 10

IARC Monographs and Technical Reports are available from the
World Health Organization Distribution and Sales, CH-1211 Geneva 27
(Fax: +41 22 791 4857)
and from WHO Sales Agents worldwide.

IARC Scientific Publications are available from
Oxford University Press, Walton Street, Oxford, UK OX2 6DP
(Fax: +44 1865 267782).

All IARC Publications are also available directly from
IARCPress, 150 Cours Albert Thomas, F-69372 Lyon cedex 08, France
(Fax: +33 72 73 83 02;
E-mail: press@iarc.fr).